Contents

Closing the
Theory–Practice Gap

A New Paradigm for Nursing

Gary Rolfe
PhD MA BSc RMN RGN NT

Principal Lecturer, School of Health Studies
University of Portsmouth, UK

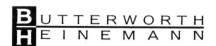

BUTTERWORTH
HEINEMANN

To Jack and Jude with love

Butterworth-Heinemann Ltd
Linacre House, Jordan Hill, Oxford OX2 8DP
A division of Reed Educational and Professional Publishing Ltd

ℝ A member of the Reed Elsevier plc group

OXFORD   BOSTON   JOHANNESBURG
MELBOURNE   NEW DELHI   SINGAPORE

First published 1996

© Reed Educational and Professional Publishing Ltd 1996

British Library Cataloguing in Publication Data
A catalogue record for this book is available from the British Library.

Library of Congress Cataloguing in Publication Data
A catalogue record for this book is available from the Library of Congress.

ISBN 0 7506 2616 X

Composition by Scribe Design, Gillingham, Kent, UK
Printed in Great Britain by Biddles Ltd, Guildford and Kings Lynn

Author and contributors

Gary Rolfe PhD MA BSc RMN PGCEA
Principal Lecturer in Research and Practice Development
School of Health Studies
University of Portsmouth

Sue Cradock SRN DipN FETC
Senior Clinical Nurse Specialist in Diabetes Nursing
Portsmouth Hospitals Trust

Melanie Jasper MSc BNurs BA RGN RHV RM NDNCert PGCEA
Principal Lecturer in Nursing Theory and Research
School of Health Studies
University of Portsmouth

Moyra Skinner SRN RMN Cert Family Therapy
Senior Nurse in Mental Health and Family Therapy
Portsmouth HealthCare Trust

Preface

Everything I say must be understood not as an affirmation but as a question

Niels Bohr

You are reading the dregs and scum of dead men

Old Chinese story

This book has evolved slowly and, in a sense, unconsciously. It has grown out of a number of journal papers published over the last 3 years on my experiences of nursing practice, research and education, and it was only in retrospect that I noticed the links between them. This is an attempt to pull them together into a coherent whole which I have perhaps overambitiously referred to as a new paradigm for nursing. I have called it a paradigm simply because I could find no other word to describe it: it is more than a model, and it is different from a model; if anything, it is perhaps a metamodel, a model *about* models, but that sounds even more ambitious and pretentious than describing it as a paradigm.

Having said that, this is not the book I wanted to write about the new paradigm. The book I wanted to write would have been an exposition of the new paradigm expressed in the language of that paradigm. However, since the paradigm does not yet exist, it has no language, at least, not one that is familiar to most nurses. Therefore, the book I have written is the first tentative description of a new paradigm expressed in the language of the old. Some critics will undoubtedly claim that I have gone too far; others (with whom I tend to agree), that I have not gone far enough. But I have gone as far as I feel able at present, given the language and concepts at my disposal.

Trying to describe something new in terms of concepts and constructs that are old and established is a difficult and thankless task, and I fear that I stand open to the accusation, as the biologist Gregory Bateson put it, of merely producing a vulgar answer to an oversimplified question; a reductionist account of a holistic philosophy. For example, I have attempted to explain the way in which expert nurses make decisions in terms of a linear, logical process, whereas my intuition and experience tells me that there is far more to it than that. I have also tried to describe a new paradigm research process as an extension of the old, whereas, in fact, I suspect that it is fundamentally different. But as the epigraph by Niels Bohr at the start of this preface has it, I am attempting to ask a question rather than to answer one; and not, I hope, an oversimplified question which produces only vulgar answers, but a naive and fundamental question which in turn will stimulate more complex questions.

There is an ancient Chinese story of a wheelwright who claimed that the books of the sages that his master was reading were merely the dregs and scum of dead men. When asked for an explanation, he gave an exposition about how the skill of making wheels could not be put into words, and that 'it must have been the same with the sages: all that was worth handing on died with them. The rest they put into books. That is why I said that you are reading the dregs and scum of dead men.'

Although this is an attempt to pass on something I believe to be worthwhile from my own experience, the charge of being the dregs and scum of a (not yet) dead man can of course be just as readily levelled at this book as at any other. However, if this book has anything to pass on, it is not the formal, static knowledge of what nursing is or should be, but a framework or paradigm through which to find out for yourself. As I said, the aim of this book is not to answer questions but to raise them.

A note on terminology

As a psychiatric nurse who was trained in the 1980s, I was brought up to eschew the medical model term 'patients' in favour of 'clients', and at the time this seemed to be a sensible move. However, I have since reconsidered: in a few cases it might still be suitable, but on the whole it does not describe the reality of the relationship between helper and helpee that exists in psychiatric (or what is now euphemistically referred to as mental health) nursing. General nursing has recently been struggling with the same issue, and has come up with 'service user' and 'customer', which I suppose reflects the spirit of the 1990s in the same way that 'client' reflected the spirit of the 1980s. However, these terms imply a parallel shift in terminology from 'nurse' to 'service provider', and after much thought, I have reverted to the term 'patient', which is used throughout this book.

I have had similar difficulties over references to gender, and whilst I fully appreciate the need for gender non-specific terminology, I have yet to come across any that is both elegant and grammatically correct, and so it is with some reluctance that I have reverted to gendered personal pronouns. Mindful of gender politics, I have employed the feminine pronoun to denote the person of power or authority in any relationship, and the masculine pronoun to denote the other; for example, a female nurse and a male patient, or a female teacher and a male student. I am also aware, however, of the dangers in stereotyping all nurses or teachers as women, and I therefore ask the reader to bear this in mind when reading the book.

Finally, I hope that my midwife and health visitor colleagues will forgive the use of the term 'nurse' throughout this book; the ideas expressed in it are intended to apply equally to midwifery and health visiting, and indeed to any interpersonal helping situation.

Gary Rolfe

Acknowledgements

No book is ever the unaided work of a single person, and this, probably more than most, owes its existence to a large number of direct and indirect influences. Firstly and most importantly, I must thank Lyn Gardner, without whose practical, emotional and intellectual support this book would never have been written.

Clearly, it would also not have been written without those friends and colleagues whose papers are included in it, but their contributions go much deeper than what appears in print. My thanks therefore go to Melanie Jasper, with whom I have collaborated on a number of research and curriculum development projects over the past 5 years; to Moyra Skinner, with whom I worked for several years, and from whom I learned an enormous amount, as part of a family therapy team; and to Sue Cradock, who has kindly involved me in her work with advanced practitioners, and who has been a tireless advocate of the ideas expressed in this book.

I also wish to thank all those friends and work colleagues who have expressed interest and given support to my work, and in particular, David Carpenter and Ian McRae, mentors, facilitators, and sometime bosses, who have both been extremely generous with their time, their ideas and their support during the 15 years that I have known them.

Thanks and sympathy must also go to the students and practitioners on whom I have tried out many of the ideas contained in this book, and who have helped to shape and modify its contents.

And lastly, I must of course thank my sons Jack and Jude for inspiration and distraction in equal measures, and to whom this book is dedicated.

Introduction

To convince someone to recognise that there may be a better way, it has to be made intelligible to them and has to be related to concepts that they already have. Not only that, but the need for a different system will not be recognised unless they can be persuaded the actual system does not work so well. For this it requires a critical examination with the resources of both science and philosophy.

A.J. Ayer

That is the way it is because it is that way
It is that way in that it is the way it is
In the way that it is is the way it is
In the way that that is the way
That is the way it is that is it is the way
Or, that it is that way is the way it is
The way it is that is the way it is
In that it is the way it is is because it is that way
Or that it is the way that it is is the way that it is that
That is the way that it is the way that it is is the way that it is that way.

Joanna Walton

The problem of the theory–practice gap

One of the most problematic and enduring issues for nursing is the observation that what happens in clinical situations rarely, if ever, matches what the textbooks say ought to happen. Most nurses will have had some experience of this so-called theory–practice gap, but it is probably felt most acutely by student nurses, who often find themselves torn between the demands of their tutors to implement what they have learnt in theory, and pressure from practising nurses to conform to the constraints of real-life clinical situations. The scenario of attempting to try out a particular technique or nursing intervention read about in a text book or research journal, only to be told 'we've already tried that and it doesn't work', or 'actually, we've found that the way we do it at the moment seems to work best' is familiar to most conscientious students eager to improve practice.

Without doubt, the problem of the theory–practice gap is the most important and fundamental issue facing the nursing profession today, since the gap between theory and practice calls into question the very foundation on which nursing is based. If nursing theory cannot account for or predict what happens in clinical practice with any degree of certainty, then the entire body of nursing knowledge is redundant and nursing is reduced to nothing more than trial and error.

Nursing theorists tell us that the theory–practice gap is between what research and theory says ought ideally to be happening, and what actually happens in the 'imperfect' clinical area. From this perspective, the problem is that nurses fail, for a variety of reasons, to make use of research findings, and the gap will only be bridged if practice moves closer to the ideals of nursing theory by nurses reading and implementing research reports. On the other hand, practitioners tell us that the gap is between what actually works in real life and the unrealistic textbook ideals. From this perspective, the gap will be bridged by nursing theory more closely reflecting the realities of clinical life. In either case:

> If it is virtually impossible for experienced nurses to relate nursing theory to everyday practice, then something is very wrong with either theory or practice. (Miller, 1985)

The fact that the gap is still very much with us suggests that neither view is an accurate representation of the actual situation, and that there is something peculiar about the relationship between theory and practice. Schön (1983) described this as a 'crisis in confidence in professional knowledge', a growing mistrust by practitioners that academic knowledge can offer anything of relevance to practice situations.

This book provides an alternative view of theory and practice which does not merely bridge the theory–practice gap, but closes it. It argues that the refusal of the gap to go away is actually a symptom of a serious underlying problem resulting from outdated theoretical concepts and a misconception about the relationship of theory to practice. The gap is a consequence of the way in which theory has failed to keep pace with changes in the concept and practice of nursing. It is an illusion, created by a way of conceptualising theory which can never fully account for what happens in clinical practice, and as such, the theory–practice gap cannot be bridged either by practice moving closer to existing theory, or by theory conforming to the constraints and limitations of real-life practice. It is a problem which must be dis-solved rather than solved, by developing a new concept of nursing theory and a new relationship between theory and practice, in which each informs and is responsive to the other.

Towards a new paradigm for nursing

Thomas Kuhn used the term 'paradigm' to describe a shared set of rules and beliefs about how a particular discipline functions. A paradigm includes 'law, theory, applications, and instrumentation together', and is 'the source of the methods, problem-field, and standards of solution accepted by any mature scientific community at any given time' (Kuhn, 1962).

The 'crisis in confidence' for nursing, highlighted by the theory–practice gap, is that current models of nursing practice no longer fit the dominant theoretical paradigm. Whereas concepts of nursing practice have undergone significant changes over the past 30 years, nursing theory, and the way that theory and knowledge are generated and disseminated, has not grown apace. Nursing theorists might espouse concepts and models of therapeutic nursing, holistic care and relationship building, but the methods they generally employ to research and teach those concepts are still based on the notion of nursing as predominantly a technical, physical care-giving activity and of patients as predictable and machine-like. In short, the dominant nursing paradigm is unsuited to the task of answering the questions posed by contemporary practising nurses.

As Kuhn has pointed out, the current paradigm influences not only theories and models of practice, but also the way in which those theories and models are generated and disseminated, that is, through research and education. In fact, theory, research and education are mutually supportive in that the prevailing models of education and research both result from, and sustain, current nursing theory, strengthening its separation from, and dominance over, practice. Nursing theory tells us that nursing is a science and that nursing knowledge is advanced through the application of scientific method. Thus, scientific research is seen as the predominant method of generating new knowledge, which strengthens the grip of science on theory, and which in turn adds weight to the scientific method, and so on.

If this vicious circle is to be broken, it can only be done so by stepping outside the dominant paradigm and initiating a radical change in the way that theory is conceptualised, implemented, formulated and disseminated, in other words, by rethinking our approach to nursing theory, practice, education and research. This involves a paradigm shift, which as Kuhn pointed out, is only likely to take place when the dominant paradigm is no longer perceived to fit reality.

The problem is that, to the naked eye, the current paradigm of nursing appears to fit very well and is growing ever stronger. After all, the 1990s have seen significant developments in nurse education, with the implementation of Project 2000 and the wholesale move of schools and colleges of nursing into higher education. In addition, there are now more research journals than ever before, and research seems to appear on every nursing agenda. Indeed, the Government recently commissioned a taskforce to examine the very subject, and its findings only served to strengthen the existing paradigm (Department of Health, 1993).

The relationship between theory, practice, research and education might appear to be well sewn up, but a closer look reveals that the seams are beginning to split. Some educationalists are beginning to question the appropriateness of Project 2000 and the traditional higher education model for the education of professionals in a practice-based discipline, and many practising nurses are starting to realise that research-based practice is not the simple process of applying research findings to practice situations that they had been led to believe.

The reasons that the current paradigm is still with us, despite strains on its seams, are firstly, that paradigms are self-perpetuating, with the generation and dissemination of knowledge within a particular paradigm only serving to strengthen that paradigm; and secondly, that paradigm shifts do not happen gradually. Mounting evidence contradicting the dominant paradigm is often denied or distorted to fit the paradigm, until it finally gives way. In the sixteenth century, the geocentric view that the Earth was the centre of the universe was stretched to breaking point to accommodate new observations which, from our perspective outside that paradigm, clearly disproved it, before it finally gave way to a new cosmology in which the Earth was seen as a minor and insignificant planet revolving around a minor and insignificant star. This involved not only a major revision of knowledge and theories about the universe, but a shift in the generation, ownership and dissemination of that knowledge and those theories, from theology to science.

Similarly, the existing paradigm of nursing has accepted the theory–practice gap as a normal and inevitable aspect of nursing life. As Kuhn pointed out, it is the scientific community of academics and researchers which decides on the problems that a discipline will recognise as legitimate, and which has the power to reject other problems 'as metaphysical, as the concern of another discipline, or sometimes as just too problematic to be worth the time' (Kuhn, 1962). Theorists have therefore either denied the significance of the theory–practice gap or else claimed that it is all the fault of practitioners for failing to implement research findings. The theory–practice gap is neither normal nor inevitable, but evidence that the current nursing paradigm of laws, theory, applications and instrumentation no longer meets the demands required of it by a new breed of holistic, patient-centred practitioners.

The aim of Part 1 of this book is to argue for a new paradigm for nursing which includes integrated models of theory, practice, research and education. Part 2 will then present working examples to demonstrate the new paradigm in action. This second part of the book contains accounts by practitioners, researchers and educators of their attempts to work with the models outlined in Part 1. It includes descriptions of practice initiatives, outlines of reflective and reflexive research methodologies, and reports of innovative curriculum development projects. This is arguably the most important part of the book, as it demonstrates the practical applications of the theoretical models and hopefully refutes the objection that they are merely theories that do not work in practice.

References

Department of Health (1993) *Report of the Taskforce on the Strategy for Research in Nursing, Midwifery and Health Visiting.* London: HMSO.

Kuhn, T.S. (1962) *The Structure of Scientific Revolutions.* Chicago: University of Chicago Press.

Miller, A. (1985) The relationship between nursing theory and nursing practice. *J. Adv. Nursing,* **10**(5), 417–429.

Schön, D.A. (1983) *The Reflective Practitioner.* London: Temple Smith.

Part 1

Towards a new paradigm for nursing

1

Nursing praxis: integrating theory and practice

It should not be forgotten that science is not the summa of life, that it is actually only one of the psychological attitudes, only one of the forms of human thought

Carl Jung

Let experience, not theory, decide upon [the practice of nursing] as upon all other things

Florence Nightingale

The changing face of nursing practice

Nursing theory has been defined as 'a logically interconnected set of propositions used to describe, explain and predict a part of the empirical world' (Riehl and Roy, 1980). This definition describes a relationship between theory and practice in which nursing theories are the key not only to understanding what happens in nursing practice, but to predict what will happen under any particular conditions. In order to understand fully how nursing theory has lost touch with the concerns of practising nurses, we must chart the changes in nursing practice over the past 40 years.

Traditional definitions of nursing have been concerned with physical care-giving and the carrying out of technical procedures in a predominantly medical setting. These definitions coincided with 'the rise of the scientific medical model dominating health care' (Wright, 1990), and reflected the traditional view of nursing as supplementary and subservient to medicine, and the traditional role of the nurse as doctor's assistant. Meleis (1985) referred to this approach to nursing as needs based, in which:

> Nursing functions were related to and determined by the needs of the patient. Physical needs were often given priority, and this tended to link the needs-based theories with the biomedical model, particularly if patient needs were related to dysfunction caused by disease or medical intervention. (Kitson, 1993)

Probably the most often quoted traditional needs based definition is that offered by Harmer and Henderson, who wrote:

> The unique function of the nurse is to assist the individual, sick or well, in the performance of those activities contributing to health or its recovery (or to peaceful death) that he would perform unaided if he had the necessary strength, will or knowledge. And to do this in such a way as to help him gain independence as rapidly as possible. (Harmer and Henderson, 1955)

This definition was, in fact, quite forward looking for its time, focusing on the *nurse assisting* the patient in the performance of activities rather than performing them herself. Other definitions of nursing care from around this time, however, have been summarised as '*doing something to or for the person* or providing information to the person with the goal of meeting needs, increasing or restoring self-help ability, or alleviating an impairment' (Marriner-Tomey, 1989, my italics). Kitson (1993) pointed out that the danger inherent in this approach to nursing is 'the ease with which nursing interventions could be reduced to a set of actions to be performed without any wider awareness of the nurse's total role in patient care'. Indeed, in the early 1970s, the majority of work in acute hospitals was still task oriented (Anderson, 1973), with the completion of tasks providing more satisfaction to nurses than patient-oriented goals (McLean, 1973). Even in the 1980s, with the move towards team nursing and patient allocation, 'nurses working in teams still tend to split care into tasks amongst the team' (Wright, 1990), and it has been observed that:

> Florence Nightingale wrote in her Notes on Nursing: 'Nursing... has been limited to signify little more than the administration of medicines and the application of poultices'. Replace the word poultice with dressing, and very little may have changed since 1859. (Schurr and Turner, 1982)

This 'task-centred' approach followed an industrial model (Lee, 1979) of breaking down care into groups of tasks, for example, the 'back round', the 'obs round' and the 'toilet round' (Wright, 1990). These activity-based, task-oriented definitions are also reflected in several nursing models, for example, Roper, Logan and Tierny's 'activities of daily living' (Roper *et al.*, 1980), which is derived directly from Harmer and Henderson's definition (Kitson, 1993), and which is largely concerned with physical nursing interventions, with assisting patients in activities that they are unable to carry out for themselves. Robinson (1993) pointed out that the vast majority of models 'had rarely been tested empirically in the practice situation', resulting in 'at best, poor science; at worst... intellectual imperialism'. Roper's model in particular has come under criticism for failing fully to account for the psychosocial needs of patients (Norman, 1987) and for identifying problems in isolation resulting in routinised care (Collister, 1988).

More recent definitions of nursing, following the example set by Peplau in the 1950s, move away from its roots in medicine and task-oriented care to focus on the importance of the individual therapeutic relationship, such that:

> an adherence to the traditions of medical science is being replaced by a professionalizing ideology for nursing, embodying holistic and person-centred approaches taking the perspective of the individual. (Bond, 1993)

This approach has been variously described as psychodynamic nursing (Peplau, 1952), humanistic nursing (Paterson and Zderad, 1976), therapeutic nursing (McMahon, 1986), primary nursing (Pearson, 1988), and patient-centred nursing (Rolfe, 1993), but more usually as psychosocial nursing. A number of descriptions and definitions from the past 25 years can be found in Table 1.1. These approaches all have different foci, but are united in their belief that 'interpersonal reactions between a patient and nurse... are often more telling in the outcome of a patient's problem than are many routine technical procedures' (Peplau, 1952). As McKee (1991) pointed out, rather than asking the nurse 'What did you do?' in a nurse–patient situation, these new ways of nursing ask 'What happened between you?'.

Table 1.1 Contemporary descriptions and definitions of nursing

---

It is one of the tasks of the professional nurse to perceive and respond to the human being in 'the patient' and to assist the ill human being in responding to the human being who is 'the nurse'. (Travelbee, 1971)

Nursing is concerned with how this particular man, with his particular history, experiences being labelled with this general diagnosis and being admitted, discharged, and living out his life with his condition as he views it in-his-world. (Paterson and Zderad, 1976)

[Nursing is] a social activity, an interactive process between individuals, the nurse and the patient. (Chapman, 1979)

Nursing involves seeing the recipient as a holistic being, and using this view to meet his or her individual needs through meaningful interaction. (Pearson, 1988)

Nursing consists of interactions between unique individuals, with unique experiences, and it always takes place in unique situations. (Sarvimaki, 1988)

Nursing is... carried out within relationships; it is, in essence, a special form of relating. (Kirby, 1995)

The contrast between the traditional and the contemporary views of nursing is graphically illustrated through the words of nursing staff who have undergone the transition. Ardern (1993) employed the technique of storytelling to access the experiences of staff on a day hospital for the elderly during the transition from a medical model to a social model of care. Reflecting on the traditional, medical model, one staff member commented that 'the orientation then was towards physical care, with the emphasis on providing a consistent routine of bathing, feeding, toileting, etc.', while another remembered that 'it was a very regimented day, you could tell the time of day by the chore or task taking place'. In contrast, nurses talking about the new model claimed that 'I feel I can offer a more varied care, giving the client the choice', 'there is more contact and counselling with relatives', and 'decisions about clients are made at ward level, not imposed by consultants'.

However, these two views of what nursing is, the traditional, task-oriented, activity-based model and the contemporary, relationship forming, holistic model, require very different methods of knowledge and theory generation, and although definitions and concepts of nursing practice have developed and moved forward over the past 40 years, the dominant paradigm for generating nursing knowledge and theories has remained unchanged.

Traditional definitions of nursing practice which focus on physical care-giving, require generalisable theories and knowledge about different treatment options at a macro, social group level. This was the view expressed at the time by professional bodies such as the RCN, which stated in 1971 that:

> To see nursing as a one-to-one relationship, even when that relationship is between the individual nurse and the individual patient, is to narrow down the concept of the nurse's role. The individual must be seen as a member of a group, and the group within the context of society. (RCN, 1971)

This macro approach to the generation of theory and knowledge, first proposed by Adam Smith in the eighteenth century, can best be provided by the scientific method and the 'generalisable and cumulative research' which the Taskforce on the Strategy for Research in Nursing (DoH, 1993) saw as being at the heart of a strategy for advancing research in nursing.

However well this model may have served in the past, with the current focus on relationship building and holistic care it is important that we understand our patients as individuals rather than as statistics. If we wish to act in the best interests of each individual patient rather than, in utilitarian terms, for the greatest good of the greatest number, then we require methods of generating theories and knowledge about 'interactions between unique individuals, with unique experiences... in unique situations' (Sarvimaki, 1988) which are accurate on a micro level rather than a macro level. The theory–practice gap, it will be argued, is a legacy of the failure of the traditional scientific paradigm[1] to account for and describe individual interpersonal relationships and a holistic view of the person.

It will be argued that the problem of the theory–practice gap is not, as theorists would have us believe, one of practice not living up to the high standards set by theory or of practising nurses failing to implement research findings, but rather that the

---

[1]Sayer (1992) has noted that there is little agreement on exactly what is meant by science apart from the fact that it is empirical, systematic and rigorous, and that disciplines such as physics and chemistry are exemplars of it. For the time being, I will restrict my use of the term to the traditional 'hard' sciences such as physics and chemistry, and the 'soft' sciences such as sociology and psychology.

whole foundation upon which nursing theory rests is inappropriate for the task of reliably informing on individual practice and individual relationships. Whilst nursing theory might not quite be, as Benner and Wrubel (1989) suggested, 'in the tradition of classical 17th Century science', it nevertheless 'maintains that a human being, like the universe, can be considered machine-like, orderly, predictable, observable and measurable'. This scientific paradigm within which nursing generally operates will now be explored in greater detail.

Science, nursing and the technical rationality model

Traditional definitions and models, following their origins in medicine, usually emphasise the scientific nature of nursing, for example: 'Nursing is a science and the application of knowledge from that science to the practice of nursing' (Andrews and Roy, 1986). This definition describes both the means by which nursing knowledge and theory is generated, and the relationship of that theory to practice. Nursing practice is determined by 'the application of knowledge' which is generated through the scientific method. And since nursing is, according to Harmer and Henderson (1955), a largely technical endeavour of doing things for other people that they are unable to do for themselves, it would seem logical to regard nursing almost as a branch of engineering, and the goal of nursing knowledge and theory as finding the most efficient and effective ways of carrying out nursing procedures.

Schön (1983) referred to this as the technical rationality model, which he described as 'the Positivist epistemology of practice', and there is little doubt that it has been spectacularly successful in the 'hard' sciences such as physics and chemistry. According to this model, science proceeds by generating hypotheses and theories to explain empirical observations, and the theory most closely resembling and explaining events in the real world is adopted. The theory is then used to make predictions, and as long as those predictions continue to coincide with reality, the theory remains in use, eventually being promoted to the status of a 'law'. However, if an existing theory no longer explains or predicts what is happening in the real world, or if a new theory emerges which more closely resembles reality, then it replaces or modifies the existing theory.

Carl Popper claimed that theories compete for acceptance in:

a process closely resembling what Darwin called 'natural selection'; that is, the natural selection of hypotheses: our knowledge consists, at every moment, of those hypotheses which have shown their (comparative) fitness by surviving so far in their struggle for existence; a competitive struggle which eliminates those hypotheses which are unfit. (Popper, 1973)

The gap between the theory and the reality which it attempts to explain therefore becomes smaller and smaller, and if theory and reality part ways, the theory is discarded. For example, Newton's theories, which seemed to explain the working of the physical world perfectly for many centuries, were finally abandoned in favour of Einstein's theories of relativity when the former were shown not to describe the real world under certain extreme conditions, such as at speeds close to that of light.

The theory-practice gap, which causes so many problems for nursing, is therefore virtually non-existent in the hard sciences, simply because the mechanism through which knowledge is generated is perfectly suited to the real world in which that knowledge is applied. In astronomy, the times of eclipses can be calculated to within a second, and in civil engineering there is an extremely close fit between the stresses and strains on a bridge predicted by theory and those found in real life. A theory-practice gap in engineering would be intolerable and totally unacceptable, and would put lives at risk. Why, then, do we continue to tolerate and accept it in nursing, where lives are equally at risk?

Even in the 'soft', social sciences[2], the gap between theory and reality is being steadily reduced. Opinion polls, for example,

[2]My distinction between 'hard' and 'soft' science is based on a rather simplistic view of hard science as characterised by invariable laws of cause and effect, such that effect E *always* follows cause C. This is contrasted with the softer social sciences which are based on the statistical techniques of correlation, and 'while the use of such techniques have (*sic*) resulted in any number of empirical generalisations, none has been so far offered as a causal law' (Hughes, 1990). When reference is made in this book to social science, I am generally referring to the positivist, quantitative school which attempts to emulate the hard sciences, rather than the interpretive, qualitative school whose aim is to construct an alternative to them. This distinction will be explored further in Chapter 2.

are becoming more and more accurate as sampling methods and questionnaire design are refined. However, whereas in a poll of voting intention it is not important to know which way each individual intends to vote, only that a certain percentage intends to vote for a certain party, in nursing the response of specific individuals is of vital importance. The reason that the theory–practice gap is being steadily reduced in the social sciences but not in nursing is because in the former, theory and reality are only required to match on a macro, statistical level, whereas in nursing it is increasingly important for theory to explain and predict on a micro, individual level. The scientific model of the relationship between theory and practice can never fully describe or account for what happens on a micro level when an individual patient encounters an individual nurse.

Although the technical rationality model has virtually eliminated the gap between theory and practice in both the 'hard' and 'soft' sciences, its success has been at the expense of a serious and substantial split between theorists and practitioners, since the natural sciences generally differentiate between the scientist or pure researcher who makes the discovery or generates the theory, and the technician or engineer who then develops its practical uses. For example, a team of scientists and researchers 'discovered' nuclear fusion, demonstrated its theoretical possibility, and outlined the conditions under which it could take place, before passing their findings to technicians who employed them to build power stations and atomic bombs. However, it is the scientists who receive the accolades for discovery, and it is the scientists whose names are remembered, not the technicians, who are viewed as little more than the scientists' assistants. Thus:

> In the evolution of every profession there emerges the researcher–theoretician whose role is that of scientific investigation and theoretical systematization. In technological professions, a division of labor thereby evolves between the theory-oriented and the practice-oriented person. (Greenwood, 1966)

When applied to nursing, the technical rationality model results in the worst of both worlds. On the one hand, the model has failed to reduce the theory–practice gap by being unable to make accurate predictions about individual care situations; and on the other hand, it has resulted in theory becoming elevated in status compared with practice, theorists becoming separated from practitioners, and research becoming something mainly carried out by the former. In addition to these drawbacks, there is no guarantee that the technical rationality model is even effective on a macro level when applied to nursing, since:

> Until well-planned evaluative research is carried out, it will be impossible to say whether it is individual skill, knowledge and sensitivity of a certain nurse or the use of a particular model which leads to the quality of care planned and given, until then we must rely on our own or others' subjective and impressionistic assessment of the benefits of using nursing models. (Webb, 1988)

Thus, even on their own positivist terms, the effectiveness of theoretical nursing models is unproven.

Nurses working under the constraints of the technical rationality model will be referred to henceforth as 'nurse–technicians', and can be seen as merely the passive implementors of theories which they had no part in developing. For example, a theorist might produce a nursing model which nurse–technicians are then expected to put into practice with their patients in their particular clinical setting, or a researcher might publish a paper demonstrating that method X is preferable to method Y in carrying out a certain procedure, leading nurse–technicians to abandon method X and adopt method Y.

This is often referred to as research-based practice, and is currently seen as an important goal for all nurses. Practising nurses have been told by the Department of Health that 'all clinical practice should be founded on up-to-date information and research findings' (DoH, 1989), but are not encouraged to engage in research themselves. The Report of the Taskforce on the Strategy for Research in Nursing, Midwifery and Health Visiting stated that:

> Many members of the nursing professions undertake small scale projects on issues which interest them.... However, it must not be seen as a substitute for the generalisable and cumulative research which we would place at the heart of a strategy for advancing research in nursing. (DoH, 1993)

This message was reinforced the following year at a conference to mark the first anniversary of the report of the Taskforce, when it was asserted that 'research, done properly, is a highly professional and specialist activity and not suited to every practitioner; but every practitioner needs to be involved in using the results of research' (DoH, 1995). Nurse-technicians are therefore being given a clear message by the Department of Health that their role is to implement the findings of others, but not to do their own research. And when nurses *do* carry out research, particularly in practice settings, it is usually dismissed disparagingly as 'project work' which is not to be confused with 'real' research, and so the schism between theorists and practitioners grows ever larger.

The problems of induction, verification and deduction

The principal tool employed by the technical rationality model for generating knowledge is the scientific method, which in its traditional form of inductivism (Hume, 1894), involves two logical mechanisms. The first is induction, whereby a finite number of individual observations are generalised into a global theory. For example, a scientist heats a test-tube of water and records the temperature at which it boils. After carrying out this experiment, say, 50 times, and finding that, each time, the water boiled at exactly 100°C, he generalises these observations into the theory that water always boils at 100°. Inductive reasoning therefore plays a significant role in theory generation. The second mechanism is deduction, whereby a global theory can be used to make predictions about individual cases. For example, the theory that water always boils at 100° can be employed to predict that the next time a test-tube of water is heated, it too will boil at 100°. Deductive reasoning therefore plays a major role in the application of global theory to individual cases. If another scientist discovers that, in the low atmospheric pressure at the top of a mountain, water actually boils at 90°, then the original theory will be discarded or modified to comply with this new view of reality, thereby ensuring an almost perfect fit between scientific theory and the real world as we currently perceive it.

Applied to nursing, this 'hard' scientific paradigm equates patients with physical, inanimate objects, and argues that just as one piece of steel will always behave in the same way as another similar piece under the same conditions, whether in a laboratory or as a component of a bridge, so too will one person always behave in the same way as another under similar conditions. Therefore, behaviour is predictable, and generalisable theories and laws of nursing are just waiting to be uncovered.

However, few nursing theorists would actually subscribe to this extreme view, and nursing research has therefore opted for the 'softer' social science paradigm rather than that of the hard, physical sciences. Whereas the paradigm of the physical sciences is based on the fact that similar objects always behave in similar ways, people are unique individuals whose behaviours and responses are, on an individual level, unpredictable. The social science paradigm therefore relies heavily on the concept of probability. It would be very unusual for a nursing research study to find that *all* the subjects responded better to one treatment method than to another. Our study might find, for example, that on average 90 per cent of all patients respond better to method X, but it will not tell us *which* 90 per cent; it is only *probable* that a certain individual patient will respond. This method of inductivism in both the hard and the soft sciences is shown in Figure 1.1.

The major problem for the hard sciences with inductivism is with the process of induction itself, since however many times an event is observed to happen, there is no logical necessity for it to continue to happen. For example, however many times our scientist observes his test-tube of water boiling at 100°, it is always possible (although, in this case, improbable) that the next time the experiment is carried out, the water might boil at 50°, or it might not boil at all, or it might freeze. This problem of induction is compounded in the soft social sciences by the fact, outlined above, that it is very unusual to produce *any* effect that occurs every time. Nine patients out of ten might respond better to treatment X, but being human and therefore unique, there will probably be at least one for whom treatment Y works better. It can be seen, therefore, that global assertions of fact in nursing are virtually impossible. We can rarely state that treatment X is *always* the best treatment, in every instance with every patient, but only that, on average, it seems to work best. Karl Popper (1963) therefore concluded that 'induction, i.e. inference based on many observations, is a myth. It is neither a psychological

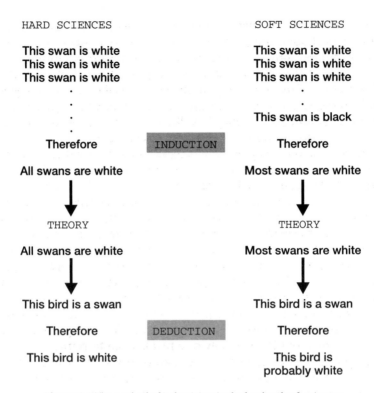

Figure 1.1 The method of inductivism in the hard and soft sciences

fact, nor a fact of ordinary life, nor one of scientific procedure.' He attempted to resolve this problem of induction in the hard sciences by arguing that scientific theories are not arrived at through the method of inductivism, but by proposing fully-formed hypotheses which are then given support by being tested under scientific conditions.

In fact, as Pratt (1978) has pointed out, this hypothetico-deductive method suffers from the same problems as inductivism, since however many times a hypothesis is confirmed through scientific experiment, there is always the possibility that, on the next occasion that it is tested, the findings will refute it. It is therefore just as impossible to prove a theory through the method of hypothetico-deductivism as it is through inductivism.

Furthermore, no matter how many cases are found which support a theory, the probability of the theory being true does not increase. The pre-Copernican theory that the sun and the stars revolve around the earth is supported every day by the observation of the sun rising in the east, travelling across the sky, and setting in the west. Yet however many times this phenomenon is observed, the theory is still false, and its repeated occurrence does not increase its chances of being true.

In fact, the only way of increasing the probability that a theory is true is by attempting to falsify it, and falsification in this case can only be achieved by making new predictions about the observed effects of the Sun and the planets moving around the Earth, and testing those. For example, how does the theory account for the retrograde movement of the stars? Eventually, if a theory is false, it will break down by failing to predict or explain observed phenomena, and will be replaced by a more feasible theory. Thus, although it is impossible to prove a theory, it is easy to disprove it, since this requires only one instance that runs counter to it. We can never prove the theory that all swans are white, since it is impossible to observe all past, present and future swans, but it takes only one black swan to refute it.

Hypothetico-deductivism, as it stands, does not readily apply to the social sciences, since as with inductivism, it is rare to find consistently occurring phenomena when dealing with people. It is difficult to set up a hypothesis of the type: 'Method X always results in effect A in all patients' without resorting to banal statements of fact, the proof of which would add little to the body of nursing knowledge. Therefore, when the hypothetico-deductive method *is* employed in nursing, the hypotheses are again based on probability, and generally take the form: 'Method X will result in effect A in 90% of patients'; or 'Method X will, on average, produce better effects than method Y'. The process of the hypothetico-deductive method in both the hard and soft sciences is shown in Figure 1.2.

Thus, the problems of induction, that no amount of positive cases ever proves a theory, and verification, that no amount of testing ever proves a theory, are partially resolved in the social sciences by employing the notion of statistical probability. In the 'hard' physical sciences, it does not matter which sample of water we use; as long as it is pure, it will boil at the same temperature as

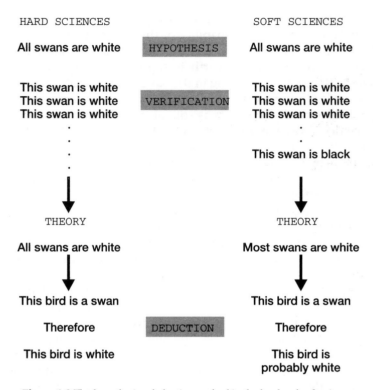

Figure 1.2 The hypothetico-deductive method in the hard and soft sciences

any other sample of pure water under the same conditions. However, because each individual person is unique and different, sampling in the social sciences is of crucial importance. The sample must represent the overall population to which we wish to generalise, but however hard we try, we can never be certain that we have selected a perfect sample which accurately reflects the population in every relevant variable.

The best we can do is to calculate the likelihood that our sample is representative, and this is referred to as the level of significance (p), which represents the probability of our research findings being contaminated due to errors in the sampling method. Degrees of probability of 1 in 100 ($p = 0.01$) or 1 in 20 ($p = 0.05$) are usually considered satisfactory, but it is the researcher who must make the decision as to the level of significance that is acceptable, that is, the degree of probability that the differences between the two methods is due to chance factors. Knowledge in the social sciences is therefore largely based on statistics: we can state the *probability* that research findings are accurate, but very rarely that they are *definitely* true.

However, the cost of resolving the problems of induction and verification is that, with no global theory which fits every case, the mechanism of deduction breaks down. The hard scientist can predict with great confidence (but not, because of the above problems, with absolute certainty) that, because water has always boiled at 100°, the next test-tube, and the one after that, will also boil at 100°. The nurse theorist, however, can only say that because nine out of ten patients respond better to treatment X, the next patient is more likely than not to also respond to treatment X. However, and this is the point, she can say absolutely nothing with confidence about how *any particular patient* will respond.

This is not a problem for disciplines such as sociology, which is largely concerned with predictions at a macro, social level. It has also not been seen as a particular problem for nursing in the past, since it is a perfectly adequate method for making general statements about the effectiveness of one treatment method over another. It can tell us, to various degrees of certainty, which nursing procedure is likely to produce the best therapeutic outcomes with the greatest number of patients, for example that the use of method X is more likely to result in better wound care for the majority of patients than method Y. However, nursing is becoming more and more concerned with individualised care and with interpersonal relationships between nurse and patient, and although the paradigm of the social sciences is useful for making general statements about probability, it is of little value in making predictions about individual patients. McCaugherty (1991) made a similar point when he wrote:

> Textbooks and lectures can only paint an incomplete and generalized picture that is divorced from practice; an average view. Rather like the average British family, who have 2.2 children and live in the middle of the Bristol Channel, the average patient is not often met.

The problem of deduction therefore causes major difficulties for nursing research, and in a profession where it is becoming more and more important to predict what will happen on an individual, micro level, it is the primary cause of the theory–practice gap. Whereas in the hard sciences, the use of the scientific method ensures that the gap between theory and reality is kept to a minimum, in nursing this theory–practice gap is showing no signs of diminishing, since the scientific, hypothetico-deductive model of research can tell us nothing about individual patients and their therapeutic encounters with individual nurses. As the biologist Gregory Bateson (1979) pointed out, 'logic and quantity turn out to be inappropriate devices for describing organisms and their interactions'. It would seem that the relationship between theory and reality which has served the hard sciences so well simply does not fit the theory and practice of nursing. What is required, then, is a new model of the relationship between theory and practice, and a new paradigm for the generation of nursing theory and knowledge — indeed, a new conception of what nursing theory and knowledge actually *is*.

Towards a theory of practice

If theory can never fully explain or predict what will happen in any individual encounter between patient and nurse, it might appear that theory is of no relevance to contemporary nursing and that the notion of research-based practice is a myth. Fortunately, there is a solution to the problem, but it involves re-formulating the concepts of nursing theory and nursing knowledge to make them compatible with contemporary definitions of nursing practice as relationship building and individualised, holistic care. It has been argued that the traditional scientific paradigm is inadequate for the task of theory generation in nursing, and that the resulting knowledge is inappropriate to a conception of nursing as being concerned with the individual rather than with the group. What is required is a body of theory which describes, explains and predicts the idiosyncrasies of individual encounters between patient and nurse, that is, a theory of practice.

The first problem in establishing a theory of practice is that the term 'theory' is itself commonly used to denote the opposite of practice, for example 'the content covered in the classroom, as opposed to the actual practice of performing nursing activities' (Polit and Hungler, 1987), or when we say 'it's all very well in theory, but will it work in practice?'. In order to develop a theory of practice, we must distinguish it from both the scientific definition of the term 'theory' referred to at the start of the chapter, and also from its everyday usage.

The study of knowledge and theory is one of the primary concerns of philosophers, and is known as epistemology. Polanyi (1962) claimed that as well as objective scientific knowledge, each individual also carried around a body of personal knowledge which is often tacit, that is, not able to be put into words. Popper (1973) referred to this as World 2 knowledge, in contrast to objective, public World 3 knowledge, whereas Bertrand Russell (1967) highlighted the difference between theoretical and practical knowledge when he distinguished between 'knowledge by description', or textbook knowledge, and 'knowledge by acquaintance', or knowledge gathered from direct experience.

A graphic example of tacit, World 2 'knowledge by acquaintance' is provided by Chuang Tzu, a Chinese philosopher who lived in the third century before Christ. He told the story of a wheelwright discussing his craft:

> In making a wheel, if you work too slowly, you can't make it firm; if you work too fast, the spokes won't fit in. You must go neither too slowly nor too fast. There must be co-ordination of mind and hand. Words cannot explain what it is, but there is some mysterious art herein. I cannot teach it to my son; nor can he learn it from me. Consequently, though seventy years of age, I am still making wheels in my old age.
> (Chuang Tzu, trans. Giles, 1926)

In nursing, Benner (1984), following the philosopher Gilbert Ryle (1963), made a similar distinction between 'knowing that' and 'knowing how', where 'knowing that' corresponds to theoretical, textbook knowledge, for example, knowing that bereavement often follows a particular course; and 'knowing how' corresponds to practical, experiential knowledge, for example, knowing how to respond to patients following a bereavement. She argued that knowing how to do something does not always require theoretical knowledge, or knowing that something is the case, and becoming an expert in practice requires the development of 'know-how', of knowledge embedded in practical experience. For example, it is possible to know how to respond to the psychological needs of a patient without knowing counselling theory, just as it is possible to ride a bicycle without knowing the theory relating to why you do not fall off.

In the field of education, Carr (1980, 1986) suggested that practice is an intentional activity located in conceptual frameworks, and as such, contains its own internal theory. This kind of theory, which corresponds to Benner's 'know-how', is not something which is applied to practice, but rather, theory is implicit *in* practice, because without it, practice degenerates into random, meaningless behaviour. This notion of internal, implicit theory explains precisely how it is possible both to ride a bicycle and to give psychological support without knowing the (external, explicit) theory, Benner's 'knowing that'. In the case of cycling, it is the internal theory which organises and co-ordinates your movements, which helps you to keep your balance, and which enables you to pedal and steer at the same time. As Bateson (1979) pointed out, 'you can ride a bicycle only after your partly unconscious reflexes acknowledge the laws of its moving equilibrium'. In the case of giving psychological support, it is the internal theory which organises and co-ordinates your thoughts, which helps you to keep your emotional equilibrium, and which enables you to think and talk at the same time.

Claiming that a nurse can give support without knowing or understanding counselling theory is not to say that it is a natural, in-built ability any more than cycling is, but rather that there is another kind of theory apart from 'knowing that', which Usher and Bryant (1989) referred to as 'informal theory'. This informal theory is not scientific in the sense of being abstract and decontextualised, but neither does it suffer from being unsystematic and intuitive. It is not only organised, but is itself an organising factor.

The relationship between informal theory and practice is rather different from that between formal, scientific theory and practice. Whereas formal theory informs and dictates to practice, in the sense that a nurse using a particular counselling model will be following a particular template or process, informal theory and practice are mutually dependant and follow a

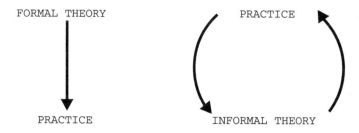

FORMAL THEORY

PRACTICE

PRACTICE

INFORMAL THEORY

Figure 1.3 The relationship between theory and practice

circular process, with practice generating theory, theory modifying practice, which generates new theory and so on (Figure 1.3). In this way, argued Schön, each practitioner builds a situational repertoire which is forever being expanded and modified to meet new situations. For example, when giving support to a patient, the nurse will draw on previous similar encounters with this or other patients, will sift through them to extract suitable interventions for the current situation, will make an appropriate response, note its effectiveness, modify it if necessary, and mentally file it away for possible later use in a similar situation.

The alternating from theory to practice to theory and so on, is so fast as to become a single integrated process, what Schön referred to as reflection-in-action, and 'it is this entire process of reflection-in-action which is central to the "art" by which practitioners sometimes deal with situations of uncertainty, instability, uniqueness and value conflict' (Schön, 1983). This 'art' is in many ways similar to what Carper (1992) referred to as aesthetic knowledge, 'knowledge of that which is individual, particular and unique', and which enables us to 'go beyond' what can be explained by scientific, empirical knowledge.

Following Schön's terminology, the nurse employing the process of reflection-in-action as a means of generating theory and knowledge in and for practice will be referred to as a 'nurse–practitioner', in contrast to the nurse–technician discussed earlier, who employs theory handed down by the theorist–scientist and adheres to the technical rationality model. The distinction made here between the nurse–technician and the nurse–practitioner is similar to that made by Elliott and Ebbutt (1985) between 'knowledge appliers' and 'knowledge generators'.

Because Schön described reflection-in-action as an art, and because it is usually unconscious, it is often mistakenly labelled as intuition, a process by which somehow the nurse mysteriously knows the right thing to do. Robinson and Vaughan (1992) referred to 'that intuitive act which makes the expert practitioner behave in an unexpected way from time to time', and Koestler provided a number of examples of major scientific discoveries where the solutions to problems appeared as 'sudden insights which seem to emerge spontaneously from the depth of the unconscious'. However, he added that:

> The moment of truth, the sudden emergence of a new insight, is an act of intuition. Such intuitions give the appearance of miraculous flashes, or short-circuits of reasoning. In fact they may be likened to an immersed chain, of which only the beginning and the end are visible above the surface of consciousness. (Koestler, 1969)

Ziman (1978) made a similar point when he described the intuitive scientist as being 'able to jump over many tedious intermediate steps, and arrive, as if by magic, at an astonishing outcome'. He stressed, however, that this sort of thinking 'merely internalises the characteristic properties and relations of concepts and operations that are already known and justifiable in public'.

Intuition is therefore not a magical process, but the unconscious workings of a prepared mind, and 'intuitive grasp should not be confused with mysticism, since it is available only in situations where a deep background understanding of the situation exists' (Benner, 1984). Benner noted that this so-called intuition was actually an important factor in contributing to expertise, by which 'expert nurses develop clusters of paradigm cases around different patient care issues, so that they approach a patient care situation using past concrete situations much as a researcher uses a paradigm' (Benner, 1984).

But it is not experience of past situations alone that results in expertise; experiences must be processed if they are to be available for reflection-in-action. The process of turning experience into knowledge is not new to most nurses, and is usually referred to as reflection or reflective practice, but is more accurately described by Schön as reflection-*on*-action. Reflection-on-action therefore provides the past paradigm cases for reflection-in-action, and the relationship between reflection-on-action and informal theory is similar to that between scientific research and formal theory. Just as the goal of the nurse–technician is research-based practice, so the goal of the nurse–practitioner is reflective practice, of reflection-in-action informed by reflection-on-action.

This is primary nursing in its truest sense, where not only is each patient responded to as an individual, in some ways similar but in many ways different from all other patients; but each individual encounter with each patient is treated as a new situation which will, in turn, modify all future encounters with all future patients. The nurse–practitioner is aware of the distinction between the disease, that is, the diagnostic label; and the illness, that is, the unique effect of a particular disease on an individual patient (Bouchier and Morris, 1982), and:

> Just as, and because, no two people are identical so no two diseases are identical; pulmonary tuberculosis, for example, in one person will be different from pulmonary tuberculosis in another (though it may bear a general resemblance), and the symptoms may vary to such an extent that it is difficult to believe that they are the same disease. (Ward, 1972)

Taking the example of mouthcare, the nurse–practitioner will draw on her situational repertoire of mouthcare interventions to find similar cases to the one she is now faced with. She will also take into account the unique situation of this individual patient, and provide care that will best meet his individual needs in a way that the nurse–technician is rarely able to do, since the technical rationality model is based on generalisable research findings which prescribe certain interventions for certain, general situations. For example, mouthcare method X might be indicated for conscious patients with dentures, mouthcare method Y for unconscious patients with their own teeth, and mouthcare method Z for unconscious patients with dentures. Although many nurse–technicians may claim to take the individual circumstances of each patient into account, they are restricted in the extent to which this is possible without undermining the principles of research-based practice and the Government strategy that 'all clinical practice should by founded on up-to-date information and research findings' (DoH, 1989). From the perspective of the technical rationality model, the nurse will have great difficulty in justifying an intervention based on what might be seen as intuition rather than on the latest research.

The nurse–practitioner, on the other hand, will be aware of the problem of deduction and the limitations of applying social science research findings to individual people. She might draw on research to help inform her decision, but her intervention will be a unique response to a unique situation rather than going 'by the book'. Informal nursing theory is therefore not generalisable in the same way that formal scientific theory tries to be. We cannot argue that because mouthcare method X proved to be better than method Y in clinical trials, then it will be better for this patient in this situation. Nevertheless, informal theory is generalisable in the sense that theory derived from reflection can be used to modify future practice. However, the relationship between theory and practice is not a deterministic or causal one, but a mutually enhancing one. Theory and practice are locked in an inseparable whole, such that reflective practice produces informal theory, which in turn modifies and develops practice.

It is as inconceivable to imagine practice without informal theory or *vice versa* as it is to imagine a magnet with a north pole but no south pole, or a coin with a head but no tail. Chinese philosophy has a particularly clear grasp of this mutually dependent relationship and expresses it through the concept of Yin and Yang, the male and female aspects of the universe, and the familiar symbol of *T'ai-chi T'u* which combines them in a 'harmonious unity' (Cooper, 1972).

Carr and Kemmis (1986) described this mutual relationship between practice and informal theory in the discipline of education:

> A 'practice', then, is not some kind of thoughtless behaviour which exists separately from 'theory' and to which it can be 'applied'.... The twin assumptions that all 'theory' is non-practical and all practice is non-theoretical are, therefore, entirely misguided.

Informal theory is contained in practice by definition, because without it practice is merely random and uncoordinated activity, and informal theory is similarly by definition generated from practice. Informal theory and practice, then, are inextricably linked, but what of formal theory? We would not wish to reject totally the influence of formal theory on practice, and we must therefore somehow integrate formal and informal theory, reflection-in-action, reflection-on-action and nursing practice into a model which fully describes and explains this new and complex relationship between theory and practice if the gap between them is ever to be closed.

Hypothetico-abductivism

We have already seen that the traditional scientific paradigm, both in the form of inductivism and of hypothetico-deductivism, is unsuitable for the construction of informal micro theory. Furthermore, the purpose of theory in traditional science is to inform and direct practice, whereas the nurse–practitioner sees theory and practice as mutually dependent and supportive. Before we can construct a new model of theory and practice for nursing, we must therefore find an alternative to the traditional scientific paradigm.

The problem with the traditional scientific method is that it was designed specifically for constructing formal, generalisable theory under more or less controlled conditions, whereas the nurse–practitioner requires informal, personal theory constructed directly from practice. The difficulty with both inductivism and hypothetico-deductivism lies in the forms of logical reasoning which they employ in going from individual instances to global theories (induction), and from global theories back to specific cases (deduction). As we saw earlier, the problem of deduction is the most difficult to resolve, since the need of the nurse–practitioner is for informal theories which describe and account for the care of individual patients rather than global theories which are unreliable on a micro level. Clearly, if we can find an alternative to inductive reasoning which avoids the necessity for constructing generalisable theories, then there is no need to employ deductive reasoning to apply those theories back to individual cases.

Although induction is, by definition, a process of generalising from specific cases to global theories, there is also a form known as specific induction or abduction, which relates to individual cases rather than to general classes. The idea of abduction is usually associated with the late nineteenth-century American philosopher Charles Pierce, who argued that it is possible to construct explanations of single events from general theories of how the world works. For example, if I know that cars require petrol in order to go, and if I observe that my car will not go, I might 'abduce' that my car has no petrol. Abductive reasoning turns formal philosophical logic on its head. A formal deductive argument might take the form:

<blockquote>
my car has no petrol;
cars need petrol in order to go;
therefore: my car will not go.
</blockquote>

Unlike in formal logic, however, in the real world we usually start with a problem (my car will not go) rather than with a premise, and we then search for a theory to explain or solve that problem. Abductive reasoning therefore begins with the conclusion and argues backwards to the premise:

<blockquote>
my car will not go;
cars need petrol in order to go;
therefore: my car has no petrol.
</blockquote>

In terms of propositional logic, this argument is flawed, since there are any number of theories that will explain this problem (no petrol, a flat battery, a broken starter motor, and so on), and so we need to apply our personal knowledge about this car in this situation in order to select the most likely theory. I might know, for example, that my car has a new battery and starter motor, but that the fuel gauge is inaccurate, and that it has been quite a while since I last filled it with petrol. The plausibility of my explanation therefore depends to a large extent on how well I am acquainted with the individual case in question, in this example, the workings of my particular car.

Having selected a formal theory as to why my car will not go (cars need petrol in order to go), based on my personal knowledge of it (it is quite a while since I last filled it with petrol), it is then possible to construct an informal theory about this particular car (my car has no petrol). It can be seen, then, that the process of abductive reasoning allows us to construct an informal theory about a specific case from a combination of formal theory and personal knowledge. It requires neither induction from the specific to the general, nor deduction from the general back to the specific, and while formal, generalisable theories are employed, they take on very much a secondary role and are tempered by personal knowledge of the specific case.

Despite its logical flaws, abductive reasoning would seem to be exactly what we are looking for in a scientific process for construction of informal, personal, micro theory, since it allows us to generate specific theories to explain individual cases from our own personal, tacit knowledge about those cases. My informal theory about why my car will not go is probably accurate, because it arose from my personal knowledge of my individual car and its unique foibles. However, as Garnham and Oakhill (1994) pointed out, 'because abductions are not deductively valid, they need to be checked', and therefore I cannot be sure that this is the true cause of the problem until I check it out by filling the car with petrol. If we phrase my informal theory of why my car will not go as a hypothesis, then filling it with petrol is a test of that hypothesis. If the car starts, the theory is confirmed; if it still will not go, then the theory is rejected and I have to look for another cause of the problem.

It should be noted, however, that the hypothesis which results from the process of abduction is not a general hypothesis about the state of the world; it is a hypothesis about an individual case, a hypothesis about my car. This combination of abductive reasoning and single case hypothesising, which we might call hypothetico-abductivism, is therefore a possible alternative to the traditional scientific paradigm for when we need to deal with individual cases in real-life situations such as primary nursing care.

Up to this point, I have employed the term 'science' to refer to the traditional scientific paradigms of inductivism and hypothetico-deductivism, but I now wish to expand that definition slightly. I am not claiming that hypothetico-abductivism is an alternative to science, but rather an *alternative scientific paradigm* to the established ones, and that entails including it within the definition of what science is. Fortunately, as Sayer (1992) has pointed out:

> there is little agreement on what kinds of methods characterise science beyond the rather bland point that it is empirical, systematic, rigorous and self-critical, and that disciplines such as physics and chemistry are exemplars of it.

Other definitions emphasise the point that science is characterised by a striving for consensus (Ziman, 1968), or that it is concerned with problem solving (Medawar, 1969). However, no single method can be said to sufficiently describe the scientific process, and 'science, no less than painting, cannot be done by numbers' (Gjertsen, 1989). Thus, there is no reason why hypothetico-abductivism should not be considered as a scientific method and as an alternative to existing scientific paradigms, since it arguably meets all of the above criteria.

Now let us take a nursing example of hypothetico-abductivism: a new patient is admitted to a psychiatric ward suffering with depression, but refuses to talk about its cause. I know that one of the causes of depression is unresolved grief following a loss (formal theory), and I suspect from my developing relationship with this patient and from my experience of similar cases (personal, tacit knowledge) that this might be his problem (informal theory). By abductive reasoning:

>   this patient is depressed;
>   unresolved grief is a cause of depression;
> therefore: this patient is suffering from unresolved grief.

Thus, from my knowledge of the formal theory that unresolved grief can cause depression, from consideration of past paradigm cases, and from my personal knowledge about the nature of this patient's depression, I can abduce the informal theory that he is suffering from unresolved grief. The accuracy of my abduction will depend on how well I know this particular patient, that is, on my personal knowledge of this individual case and of similar cases. My informal theory that this patient is depressed because he is suffering from an unresolved grief reaction can now be phrased as a hypothesis and verified or disproved by testing out predictions arising from it, for example, by exploring issues of loss with the patient. This process is summarised in Figure 1.4.

But because people are more complex than cars, the process does not end there. Having established that the patient is suffering from an unresolved grief reaction, we now need to discover what is preventing its resolution. I know that one reason for unresolved grief is that the person becomes stuck in the denial stage of bereavement, and I suspect from my relationship with this patient that this might be his problem. Therefore, from the formal theory that denial can cause unresolved grief and my personal observations and knowledge that this patient is suffering from unresolved

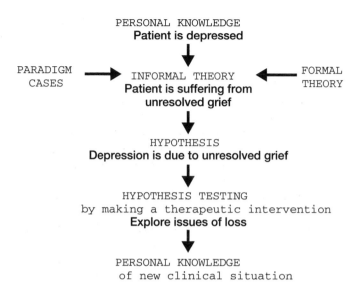

Figure 1.4 The method of hypothetico-abductivism in nursing

grief, I abduce the informal theory that he is stuck in the denial stage of bereavement. Once again, I can test hypotheses derived from this theory, which tells me even more about this particular patient and helps me to refine the problem further.

It can be seen, then, that this process of abduction and hypothesis testing can continue indefinitely, producing more and more detailed and specific theories about this patient, and that the accuracy of my hypotheses depends on the personal knowledge which I bring to the situation, and on the depth and strength of my relationship with the patient. More importantly, however, the process brings together theory and practice as part of an inseparable whole, since in testing the hypotheses which result from my theories, I must necessarily make a therapeutic intervention with my patient.

Nursing praxis

Having described an alternative scientific paradigm for the construction of informal theory, it is now necessary to examine

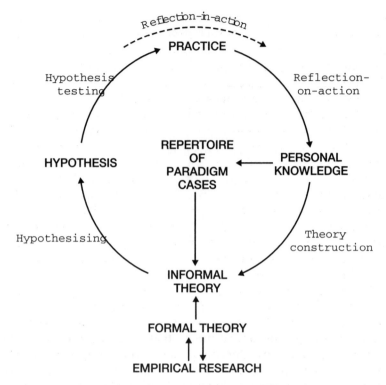

Figure 1.5 A model of nursing praxis

how it can be translated into a model of nursing to include the processes of reflection-in-action and reflection-on-action which are central to the work of the nurse–practitioner. Such a model, which will be referred to as 'nursing praxis', is shown in Figure 1.5. The term praxis was adopted by Marx to denote 'the unity of theory and practice', but it has its roots in Ancient Greece, where Aristotle used it to describe a particular form of 'doing action' employed in the practical sciences.

At the heart of the model of nursing praxis described here is the method of hypothetico-abductivism, which as we have seen, is a coming together of theory and practice involving a process of hypothesising and testing out informal theory, and modifying practice according to the results. Nursing praxis begins with reflection-on-action, which except with very experienced practitioners, involves thinking about and analysing practice situations after the event and away from the clinical area. The outcome of reflection-on-action is personal knowledge about specific situations, which can be stored away for later use as paradigm cases, or which can be employed immediately in the construction of informal theory.

Informal theory is created through the process of abductive reasoning, from a combination of personal knowledge about the patient, paradigm cases of similar situations, and formal theory from nursing or one of the supporting disciplines such as sociology, psychology or biology. The resulting informal theory is very different from formal theory. Informal theory is context specific, referring *to this* patient in *this* situation, and exists only in relation to practice, since it must be tested out in real situations before it can be accepted. Formal theory, on the other hand, refers to global situations and exists independently of practice, standing in a hierarchical relationship to it.

Having constructed an informal theory about a specific clinical situation, the next stage is to form and test a hypothesis derived from it. This involves making predictions about the outcome of specific interventions based on the theory, trying out the interventions with the patient, and noting whether the predicted outcome occurs. If it does, not only has an informal theory been constructed and tested, but a clinical intervention based on that theory has been implemented, and it is in this sense that nursing praxis can be said to integrate theory and practice into an inseparable whole.

Having tested her theory in practice, the nurse–practitioner now has two options. She can engage in further reflection-on-action in order to increase her body of personal knowledge, which in turn can be employed in more theory development. However, this will entail waiting for an opportunity to sit down away from the clinical area in order to reflect on her experience. Alternatively, she could attempt to engage in the process of reflection in the clinical area in direct and immediate response to the changes in practice she has implemented.

This is reflection-in-action, and involves a cyclical process of theory modification and hypothesis testing as part of clinical practice. It is also known, for obvious reasons, as on-the-spot experimenting, and bears a close relationship to the learning cycle described by Kolb and Fry (1975) of experience, observation and reflection, generalisation and conceptualisation, and active experimentation. Because it is a cyclical process involving both theory and practice, reflection-in-action is not only reflective, but also reflexive. Theory is tested by modifying practice, but practice also changes theory in a virtuous circle. Theory and practice are therefore developing in direct response to one another in a process which can continue indefinitely.

In order to see how nursing praxis works, let us take the example of a terminally ill patient who asks the nurse if he is dying. There are many possible reasons why a patient might ask such a question, ranging from a need for factual information to a need for reassurance that he is not dying, and it is imperative that the nurse–practitioner understands the unique needs of this individual patient in formulating her response. Her decision on how to respond will therefore be based primarily on her personal knowledge of this patient, gained from her previous reflection-on-action, but will also draw on paradigm cases from similar situations with other patients.

Although this personal knowledge will provide the main factors in coming to a decision, she may also take from formal theory in the form of principles of counselling or humanistic psychology, theories of ethical behaviour, and experimental research. However, these considerations will be secondary, they will provide a range of options for the generation of an informal theory about this patient in this situation, and will inform her practice rather than direct it.

Having constructed an informal theory about this patient, his reasons and motives for asking whether he is dying, and the most effective response, the nurse–practitioner now tests out a hypothesis based on that theory by responding to the patient and assessing the impact of her response. Her informal theory might, for example, be that this patient genuinely wants to know whether he is dying in order to put his mind at rest, and also that he is psychologically equipped to deal with the consequences of being told. Her hypothesis in this case would be that, if the information is given in a caring, sensitive and supportive manner, his anxiety and distress would reduce on being told. Having made her intervention, the nurse–practitioner then continues around the cycle again by making a new assessment of the transformed clinical situation, that is, whether or not the patient's anxiety has reduced, generating further personal knowledge, and so on.

Let us now take a real-life case. Benner (1984) provided a great many examples in her book *From Novice to Expert* of what she referred to as expert practice. The following extract, recounted by an Intensive Care Unit nurse, was used by Benner to illustrate how an expert is able to succinctly describe an emergency situation, but it is also an excellent, if unwitting, account of nursing praxis and the process of hypothetico-abductivism.

> I had worked late and was just about ready to go home, when a nurse preceptor said to me, "Jolene, come here". Her voice had urgency in it, but not Code Blue. I walked in and I looked at the patient and his heart rate was about 120, and he was on the respirator and breathing. And I asked her: "what's wrong?". There was a new graduate taking care of him. And he just pointed down to the patient who was lying in a pool of blood. There was a big stream of blood drooling out of his mouth. The man's diagnosis was mandibular cancer which had been resected, and about a week previous to that he had had a carotid bleed from the external carotid which had been ligated secondary to radiation erosion. That wound had become septic and he had developed respiratory failure and he was in ICU for that. So I looked at the dressing and it was dry, the blood was coming out of his mouth. The man had a tracheostomy because of the type of surgery that had been done. He also had an N.G. tube for feedings, and I got to thinking that it might be the innominate or the carotid artery that had eroded. So we took him off the ventilator to see if anything was going to pump out of the trach. There was a little blood, but it looked mostly like it had come down from the pharynx into the lungs. So we began hand ventilating him, trying to figure out what the devil was inside his mouth that was pumping out this tremendous amount of blood.... (Benner, 1984)

It can be seen from this account that the nurse employed a combination of formal theory of anatomy and personal knowledge of this patient in order to construct the informal theory that the patient was bleeding from an eroded carotid artery. She then tested her hypothesis by taking the patient off the ventilator and, we are told by Benner, applying pressure to the carotid artery. This action confirmed the hypothesis and resolved the immediate problem, and the nurse now turned her attention to the patient's lowered blood pressure, which presented a new set of problems to solve.

This example demonstrates that the model of nursing praxis, which forms the foundation of a new paradigm of nursing, describes the process by which some, and perhaps many, nurses already make clinical decisions, particularly since reflective practice is rapidly becoming an everyday feature of nursing in a wide variety of settings. It might be objected that we do not need what appears to be a complex explanation for a natural and simple process, and that nurses will continue to practise in this way whether or not it is formalised as a model of nursing. However, it is important that nurses can describe and justify what they do, and are able to refute charges that they are working by trial and error. Furthermore, the model has profound implications for practice, as well as exerting an influence on education and research, and an example of working in this way will be given in Part 2 of this book.

Nursing praxis and the nurse–practitioner

In order to appreciate fully the implications of the role of the nurse-practitioner, it will be contrasted with the traditional nurse-technician role. It should be borne in mind that we are talking about what Weber (1946) referred to as ideal types, the 'perfect' cases of the two roles which are rarely found in real-life situations. The ideal type nurse-technician is committed to research-based practice, that is, her clinical decisions are based to a great extent on public, generalisable knowledge generated through research either in nursing or in one of the supporting disciplines such as psychology, sociology or biology. This knowledge is, on the whole, obtained through reading journals and books, or from attending lectures, Russell's 'knowledge by description', and will constitute a shared ethos of practice comprised of a body of theories and models. The nurse-technician will use intervention X in situation A because it has been found through research to be the most effective form of intervention in the majority of cases. Nursing interventions are therefore procedural, and are based on a consensus of shared theory and knowledge throughout the profession.

The ideal type nurse-practitioner, on the other hand, is committed to reflective practice. Her clinical decisions are based to a great extent on private, tacit, personal knowledge, Russell's 'knowledge by acquaintance', a situational repertoire generated through the process of reflection-on-action and reflection-in-action. Personal knowledge of this sort cannot be passed on from one person to another, and theory is constructed by what Schön referred to as on-the-spot experimenting, by which the nurse–practitioner, when faced with a new situation, draws on her personal knowledge and experience to construct a hypothesis, acts on that hypothesis, evaluates the effectiveness of the intervention, modifies the hypothesis, refines the intervention, re-evaluates, and so on, in a continuous cycle.

The main difference between the nurse-technician and the nurse-practitioner, therefore, is that whereas the former bases her practice on public, shared theories and knowledge, the latter generates her own theory out of her own practice, and applies it back to that practice. The theory-practice gap is therefore abolished: since theory and practice are simply two faces of the same coin of nursing praxis, there is not even the concept of a gap. When the nurse-technician uses intervention X in situation A, there is always the chance, due to the problem of deduction, that patient P will respond whereas patient Q will not. However, when the nurse-practitioner uses intervention Y in situation A with patient P, she knows that the patient will respond because intervention Y was developed through a process of on-the-spot experimenting with patient P, and is therefore tailored precisely to patient P's personal needs. Tomorrow, patient P may present a different situation requiring a different intervention, and the nurse-practitioner will not automatically assume that because intervention Y was successful with patient P that it will work with everyone in every situation, or even with the same patient in different situations. She will go through the process of on-the-spot experimenting in each new encounter, and next time she might respond with intervention Y again, or she might respond with intervention Z.

So where do the academic and the theorist fit into the picture? The nurse-practitioner does not reject public, research-based models and theories, but merely wishes to place them in their true context. The most important and relevant knowledge and theories on which to base clinical decisions are those generated by the practitioner herself out of her own practice. However, objective, World 3 knowledge can be employed to inform and support clinical decisions and clinical practice, as in the example described earlier, where the response to a dying patient was based primarily on personal knowledge and reflection-in-action, but also drew on principles of counselling or humanistic psychology, on ethical considerations, and on experimental research.

By generating theories and knowledge through reflection-on-action and on-the-spot experimenting, the nurse–practitioner is also a researcher. This role of practitioner-as-researcher does not fit the traditional model of the nurse researcher as a specialist, coming into the clinical area to 'do' research. In fact, the role of researcher cannot be separated from the role of practitioner, because to practise is to research, although this research will not conform to the technical rationality model, in which findings from large samples are generalised to whole populations. Indeed, the kind of research which the nurse–practitioner engages in might have a sample of one, and might not be generalisable beyond that single person. Nevertheless, it is still research, and not subject to the same problems of induction and deduction as positivist scientific research. More importantly, it does not contribute to the widening of the theory–practice gap. This new model of nursing research will be discussed in greater depth in the following chapter.

As well as the role of the researcher, the traditional role of the nurse educator is also under threat from the nurse–practitioner. The nurse–practitioner is more concerned with tacit, personal knowledge and informal theories than with general, universal, formal theories, since nurse-patient encounters and relationships are constantly developing and changing and no single theory can account for the complexities of any given situation. Education for the nurse–practitioner is therefore less a transmission of knowledge from teacher to pupil than a facilitation of theory and knowledge generation by the nurse herself. Lectures and other formal teaching methods will have little relevance, and will be replaced by group work, role-play, reflective diaries and critical incident analysis.

Furthermore, although the classroom might be a suitable place to reflect on experience, the real business of theory and knowledge construction will occur in the practice setting during actual clinical work. The nurse teacher clearly has a limited role to play in this setting; the traditional clinical teacher, who comes into the practice area to demonstrate expert practice will be redundant, since expertise can only be acquired through repeated experience. The nurse–practitioner will be the expert at nursing practice, and the teacher will have to develop expertise in the practice of education as the facilitation of reflection. Nurse education will therefore be an encounter between equals, between the experienced practitioner and the experienced educationalist. The role of the teacher will not be to teach nursing, an impossible task from the perspective of the model of nursing praxis, but to facilitate the practitioner to convert her experience into expertise through reflection-on-action and reflection-in-action. This new approach to education will be discussed in detail in Chapter 3, and an example of how one teacher has responded to the challenge that this approach raises will be outlined in Part 2.

The most significant consequence of this shift in importance from research-based knowledge to experiential knowledge and praxis is that the status of nursing practice and the ward-based, clinical nurse is elevated in accordance with her new role as researcher and generator of theory. She no longer merely applies theories dictated by educationalists and researchers; she is an educationalist and a researcher. In short, the nurse–practitioner is an expert with 'a deep background understanding of clinical situations based upon many past paradigm cases' (Benner, 1984).

Many nurses will claim, while continuing to support the technical rationality model and the notion of research-based practice, that of course they respond to patients as individuals and tailor their interventions to the specific and unique needs of each person. This is undoubtedly true, but what it demonstrates is not the adequacy of the technical rationality model, but its inability to provide appropriate and effective interventions on a micro level. By moving towards nursing praxis, the nurse–technician is expressing her dissatisfaction with a paradigm that is woefully inadequate to the task of equipping her to give the best and most effective care to each individual patient. She is saying, in effect, 'yes, I will continue to pay lip service to research-based practice, I will continue to work on the assumption that research can provide answers on an individual level, but in the cases where it doesn't work, I will ignore it and base my clinical decisions on my own experience instead'. Feyerabend made a similar point when he wrote:

> Everywhere science is enriched by unscientific methods and unscientific results while procedures which have often been regarded as essential parts of science are quietly suspended or circumvented. (Feyerabend, 1978)

Schön has described this discrepancy as between espoused theories, those theories that practitioners claim to base their practice on, and theories-in-use, those theories that they actually employ in real life. With the move towards primary nursing and individualised patient care, nurses have very quickly run up against the limitations of a paradigm which, in the words of Aggleton and Chalmers (1986), is 'dehumanising the process of nursing by drawing an analogy between a human being and a machine', and are finding their own solutions. The current paradigm is failing nurses and patients, and needs to be replaced; the model of nursing praxis and the role of the nurse–practitioner are the foundations of a new paradigm for nursing which addresses the needs and requirements of the modern nurse.

References

Aggleton, P. and Chalmers, H. (1986) *Nursing Models and the Nursing Process*. London: Macmillan.

Anderson, E.R. (1973) *The Role of the Nurse*. London: Royal College of Nursing.

Andrews, H.A. and Roy, C. (1986) *Essentials of the Roy Adaptation Model*. Norwalk: Appleton-Century-Crofts.

Ardern, P. (1993) *The Introduction Of A Social Psychological Model Of Care Into A Day Hospital For Dementia Sufferers*. Unpublished Dissertation, University of Portsmouth.

Bateson, G. (1979) *Mind and Nature*. London: Fontana.

Benner, P. (1984) *From Novice to Expert*. California: Addison-Wesley.

Benner, P. and Wrubel, J. (1989) *The Primacy of Caring*. California: Addison-Wesley.

Bond, S. (1993) Experimental research in nursing: necessary but not sufficient. In: Nursing: Art and Science (A. Kitson, ed.) London: Chapman and Hall.

Bouchier, I.A.D. and Morris, J.S. (1982) *Clinical Skills*. London: Saunders.

Carper, B. (1992) Philosophical inquiry in nursing: an application. In: *Philosophic Inquiry in Nursing* (J.F. Kikuchi and H. Simmons, eds) Newbury Park: Sage.

Carr, W. (1980) The gap between theory and practice. *Journal of Further and Higher Education*, 4(1), 60-69.

Carr, W. (1986) Theories of theory and practice. *Journal of Philosophy of Education*, 20(2), 177-186.

Carr, W. and Kemmis, S. (1986) *Becoming Critical*. London: Falmer Press.

Chapman, C. (1979) Sociological theory related to nursing. In: *Readings in Nursing* (M.M. Colledge and D. Jones, eds) Edinburgh: Churchill Livingstone.

Chuang Tzu (translated by H.A. Giles) (1926) *Chuang Tzu*. London: George Allen and Unwin.

Collister, B. (1988) *Psychiatric Nursing*. Using Models of Nursing Series. London: Edward Arnold.

Cooper, J.C. (1972) *Taoism: the Way of the Mystic*. Wellingborough: The Aquarian Press.

Department of Health (1989) *A Strategy for Nursing: A Report of the Steering Committee*. London: DoH.

Department of Health (1993) *Report of the Taskforce on the Strategy for Research in Nursing, Midwifery and Health Visiting*. London: HMSO.

Department of Health (1995) *The Nursing and Therapy Professions' Contribution to Health Services Research and Development*. London: DoH.

Elliott, J. and Ebbutt, D. (1985) *Issues in Teaching for Understanding*. Harlow: Longmans, for Schools Council.

Feyerabend, P. (1978) *Science in a Free Society*. London: New Left Books.

Garnham, A. and Oakhill, J. (1994) *Thinking and Reasoning*. Oxford: Blackwell.

Gjertsen, D. (1989) *Science and Philosophy*. Harmondsworth: Penguin.

Greenwood, E. (1966) Attributes of a profession. In: *Professionalization* (H.M. Vollmer and D.L. Mills, eds) Englewood Cliffs: Prentice-Hall.

Harmer, B. and Henderson, V. (1955) *Textbook of the Principles and Practice of Nursing*. New York: Macmillan.

Hughes, J. (1990) *The Philosophy of Social Research*. London: Longman.

Hume, D. (1894) (First published in 1748 under a different title) *A Treatise of Human Nature* (L.A. Selby-Bigge, ed.). Oxford: Clarendon Press.

Kirby, C. (1995) The world of nursing. In: *Theory and Practice of Nursing* (L. Basford and O. Slevin, eds) Edinburgh: Campion Press.

Kitson, A. (1993) *Nursing: Art and Science*. London: Chapman and Hall.

Koestler, A. (1969) *The Act of Creation*. London: Picador.

Kolb, D.A. and Fry, R. (1975) Towards an applied theory of experiential learning. In: *The Theories of Group Processes* (C.L. Cooper, ed.) London: John Lilley and Sons.

Lee, M.E. (1979) Towards better care: primary nursing. *Nursing Times*, **75**(33), 133–135.

Marriner-Tomey, A. (1989) *Nursing Theorists and their Work*. St Louis: C.V. Mosby.

McCaugherty, D. (1991) The theory–practice gap in nurse education: its causes and possible solutions. *J. Adv. Nursing*, **16**, 1055–1061.

McKee, C. (1991) Breaking the mould: a humanistic approach to nursing practice. In: *Nursing as Therapy* (R. McMahon and A. Pearson, eds) London, Chapman and Hall.

McLean, J.P. (1973) Nursing care study: bilateral nephrectomy. *Nursing Mirror*, **136**(10), 31–34.

McMahon, R.A. (1986) Nursing as therapy. *Professional Nurse*, **1**(10), 270–272.

Medawar, P. (1969) *The Art of the Soluble*. Harmondsworth: Penguin.

Meleis, A. (1985) *Theoretical Nursing: Development and Progress*. Philadelphia: Lippincott.

Norman, A. (1987) *Severe Dementia: The Provision of Long Stay Care*. London: Centre of Policy on Aging.

Paterson, J.G. and Zderad, L.T. (1976) *Humanistic Nursing*. New York: Wiley.

Pearson, A. (1988) *Primary Nursing*. London: Croom Helm.

Peplau, H.E. (1952) *Interpersonal Relationships in Nursing*. Basingstoke: Macmillan.

Polanyi, M. (1962) *Personal Knowledge: Towards a Post-critical Philosophy*. London: Routledge and Kegan Paul.

Polit, D.F. and Hungler, B.P. (1987) *Essentials of Nursing Research: Methods and Applications*. Philadelphia: Lippincott.

Popper, K.R. (1963) *Conjectures and Refutations*. London: Routledge and Kegan Paul.

Popper, K. R. (1973) *Objective Knowledge: an Evolutionary Approach*. Oxford: OUP.

Pratt, V. (1978) *The Philosophy of the Social Sciences*. London: Routledge.

Riehl, J.P. and Roy, C. (1980) *Conceptual Models for Nursing Practice*. New York: Appleton-Century-Crofts.

Robinson, J. (1993) Problems with paradigms in a caring profession. In: *Nursing: Art and Science* (A. Kitson, ed.) London: Chapman and Hall.

Robinson, K. and Vaughan, B. (1992) *Knowledge for Nursing Practice*. Oxford: Butterworth Heinemann.

Rolfe, G. (1993) The Patient-centredness Multi-choice Questionnaire: developing an instrument for the measurement of patient-centredness in student nurses. *J. Adv. Nursing*, **18**, 120–126.

Roper, N., Logan, W.W. and Tierney, A.J. (1980) *The Elements of Nursing*. Edinburgh: Churchill Livingstone.

Royal College of Nursing and National Council of Nurses of the United Kingdom (1971) *RCN Evidence to the Committee on Nursing*. London: RCN.

Russell, B. (1967) *The Problems of Philosophy*. Oxford: OUP.

Ryle, G. (1963) *The Concept of Mind*. Harmondsworth: Penguin.

Sarvimaki, A. (1988) Nursing as a moral, practical, communicative and creative activity. *J. Adv. Nursing*, **13**, 462–467.

Sayer, A. (1992) *Method in Social Science*. London: Routledge.

Schön, D.A. (1983) *The Reflective Practitioner*. London: Temple Smith.

Schurr, M.C. and Turner, J. (1982) *Nursing — Image or Reality*. London: Hodder and Stoughton.

Travelbee, J. (1971) *Interpersonal Aspects of Nursing*. Philadelphia: F.A. Davis.

Usher, R. and Bryant, I. (1989) *Adult Education as Theory, Practice and Research*. London: Routledge.

Ward, F.A. (1972) *A Primer of Pathology*. London: Butterworth.

Webb, C. (1988) Organising care, nursing models a personal view. *Nursing Practice*, **1**, 208–212.

Weber, M. (1946) *From Max Weber: Essays in Sociology*. London: Routledge and Kegan Paul.

Wright, S.G. (1990) *My Patient — My Nurse*. London: Scutari.

Ziman, J. (1968) *Public Knowledge*. Cambridge: Cambridge University Press.

Ziman, J. (1978) *Reliable Knowledge*. Cambridge: Cambridge University Press.

2

Research for nursing praxis

Truths are illusions which one has forgotten are illusions

Friedrich Nietzsche

Where is the wisdom we have lost in knowledge?
Where is the knowledge we have lost in information?

T.S. Eliot

Nursing research and the social science paradigm

It was argued in the previous chapter that nursing adopted the paradigm of the social sciences at a time when nursing practice was seen as task oriented and as subservient to medicine, and when nursing theory was attempting to achieve scientific credibility to support that view of practice. However, as nursing practice developed to become separate and autonomous from medicine, and concerned with individual therapeutic relationships, nursing theory failed to keep pace, resulting in a body of theory which could no longer explain or predict the new concerns of practice such as relationship building and one-to-one encounters between patient and nurse.

This schism between theory and practice is very apparent in nursing research, where the vast majority of definitions and explanations of the process and purpose of research no longer reflect the current concerns of practice. A selection of definitions of nursing research can be found in Table 2.1.

These definitions all make virtually the same point, that research employs the scientific method in order to increase knowledge, facts and theories. There is hardly any mention of

Table 2.1 Definitions of nursing research

[Research is] a planned, systematic search for information, for the purpose of increasing the total body of man's (*sic*) knowledge. (Lancaster, 1975)
[Research is] an attempt to identify facts, and the relationship between and among facts, by systematic, scientific enquiry in order to increase available knowledge. (Hunt, 1982)
The major reasons for doing research in nursing are providing the profession with a body of scientific knowledge and identifying and developing nursing theories. (Treece and Treece, 1986)
The primary goal of nursing research is to develop a scientific knowledge base for nursing practice. (Burns and Grove, 1987)
[Research is] an attempt to increase available knowledge by the discovery of new facts or relationships through systematic enquiry. (Clark and Hockey, 1989)
[Research is] rigorous and systematic enquiry... designed to lead to generalisable contributions to knowledge. (Department of Health, 1993)

practice, and where it is referred to, it is seen as dependent on the generation of knowledge. The reason that practice development is not seen as a legitimate goal of nursing research in its own right is because the social science paradigm within which nursing research is situated views the goal of research as the development of theory rather than practice. For example, May claimed that:

> Social theory is not something which can be separated from the process of social research. Theory informs our thinking which, in turn, assists us in making research decisions and sense of the world around us. Our experiences of doing research and its findings, in its turn, influences our theorizing; there is a constant relationship that exists between social research and social theory. (May, 1993)

Furthermore, as Sayer pointed out:

> Social scientific knowledge is primarily propositional or referential, rather than practical, and this should immediately provide some clues as to why it seems unable, except very indirectly, to help us decide how to live. (Sayer, 1992)

The way that research is conducted in the social sciences is largely dependent on the researcher's beliefs about the nature and purpose of social knowledge and theory. Most writers accept that there are two dominant models of research in the social sciences, which reflect two different and diverse views of social reality, such that 'the two traditions reflect fundamentally different epistemologies concerning the sort of knowledge about the social world which it is possible to achieve and different philosophies as to the nature of man' (Walker, 1985). Sarantakos (1994) referred to them as positivist and interpretive, Cohen and Manion (1985) as positivist and anti-positivist, and Harré (1979) as extensive and intensive, where in each case the former employs mainly quantitative methodologies, and the latter employs mainly qualitative methodologies.

Nursing has joined the debate rather late in the day, and many nurse–researchers purport to see beyond the dichotomy and advocate 'what might be termed methodological pluralism and pragmatism' (Bond, 1993), which not only argues that the research method should be selected to fit the question being asked, but that several diverse methods could be employed in the same study. Furthermore, 'quantitative and qualitative research methods complement each other, because they generate different kinds of knowledge that are useful in nursing practice' (Burns and Grove, 1987), and 'often the strongest research findings are in studies that utilise both methods' (Field and Morse, 1985).

In nursing research, unlike in the social sciences, the positivist and interpretive schools 'are in fact just two different approaches to data collection and analysis and not two different philosophies of life' (Chapman, 1991). In fact, nursing research has largely subsumed the qualitative methodologies under the positivist, technical rationality model, and whereas a great many nursing research projects employ a qualitative approach, it is usually within the dominant model of technical rationality. For example, Janice Morse, a leading qualitative nurse–researcher, observed that:

> Qualitative methods came into nursing through nurses who, while participating in the Nurse Scientist Program, obtained their doctorate in other fields, such as anthropology. When these *scientists* returned to nursing, they continued to conduct research using the methods of their adopted discipline. (Morse, 1991, my italics)

Morse clearly identifies qualitative research with science, and the extent to which the traditional scientific paradigm has influenced nursing research can be seen from all the definitions of nursing research in Table 2.1.

This model sees scientific enquiry as being founded on strict rules and procedures; as being generalisable; as being based on universal laws of causation; and as being neutral and value-free. It emphasises the collection and analysis of largely quantitative data, and although many nurse–researchers utilise qualitative methodologies, they usually do so from within a far more rigorous scientific framework than their colleagues in the social sciences. Furthermore, inductive research such as single case studies or small-scale phenomenological studies are given little support by the majority of nursing research funding bodies.

It was argued in Chapter 1 that the technical rationality model has also contributed to the separation of theory from practice in nursing and the widening of the theory-practice gap by suggesting that nursing is advanced through the generation of knowledge and theories by academics and researchers, which are then applied by nurses in much the same way as academics and scientists developed the theory of atomic fission, which was then applied by technicians to making bombs and building power stations. A distinction is created between 'knowledge appliers' and 'knowledge generators' (Elliott and Ebbutt, 1985), and the nurse is cast in the former role of technician to the theoretician's role of scientist. It is therefore the nurse–technician who is usually blamed for the subsequent failure of much nursing theory to be successfully applied to practice, through either not being aware of current research findings or not properly implementing them. For example, Chapman observed that:

> In the author's experience, when questioning groups of nurses at the beginning of a research course/lecture as to the professional reading they had undertaken in the preceding week many will admit to having looked at the weekly journals only. On further questioning the respondents tend to identify that, within these journals, the news pages and the job advertisements have received attention and few are able to recount the content or even the subject matter of any research reports contained in the journal. (Chapman, 1991)

Chapman supported this observation by reference to two studies which were both over 10 years old at the time she was writing, and it is rather worrying that an author criticising practising nurses for not valuing scientific research should be offering such unscientific 'evidence' as anecdotes and out of date studies for her assertion.

Another reason given by Chapman for the theory–practice gap is nurses' 'unwillingness to accept research findings which directly challenge traditionally held beliefs and practices.... The disbelief of the findings is a defence for the accepted practice' (Chapman, 1991). However, what Chapman fails to consider is that the traditionally held beliefs which she accuses nurses of being unwilling to give up are themselves often based on earlier research findings, which were promoted by researchers and theorists as fact or truth with as much vigour as they are now promoting their latest version of the truth. In their enthusiasm to have their current research findings accepted and implemented, researchers are failing to acknowledge and communicate the provisional nature of all research-based knowledge.

It was also argued in the previous chapter that the theory–practice gap is not a result of the failure of practising nurses to read or implement research findings, but rather that most nursing research is carried out from within a theoretical framework unsuited to current nursing practice, and is therefore impossible to apply successfully, since generalisable, deductive findings have little meaning in individual interpersonal nurse–patient situations. This argument is supported by the observations of MacGuire (1991), who pointed out:

> not all nurses who engage in patient care fully accept the arguments for research-based practice. Many do not feel that research necessarily has relevance to their own work and fail to see a role for themselves in the development of practice through research. Research, for a variety of reasons, has not always addressed the concerns of clinical nurses and frequently does not produce the kind of reliable guide to practice that practitioners require.

Thus, rather than advancing nursing, most current research is, in fact, holding it back by failing to address the real needs of nurse–practitioners at a micro level. But if nursing is not advanced through the generation of knowledge and theories using the scientific method, then what has research to offer nursing?

Nursing research and the problem of deduction

If research is to be defined along the narrow parameters of the positivist, scientific, technical rationality model, then the answer to the above question would have to be: very little. The aim of the traditional scientific model of research is to generate knowledge and build theory, either by inductivism or hypothetico-deductivism, which is then applied, through the process of deduction, to practice situations (Figure 2.1). But whereas in the 'hard' sciences such as physics and chemistry each individual subject, say a test-tube of water, will behave in the same way; and whereas in the 'soft' sciences such as sociology it is rarely necessary to make statements about individual cases at all, in nursing each individual encounter between nurse and patient is not only important, but is different and unique.

Heisenberg (1963) observed that even in the hard sciences, the behaviour of matter is unpredictable at the sub-atomic level, but this is precisely where physics and positivist sociology share similarities which nursing does not. Physical material is unpredictable on a micro, sub-atomic level, but almost perfectly predictable at the macro, 'physical' level at which most practical work is done, for example in estimating the tensile strength of steel. Social 'material' is unpredictable on a micro, individual person level, but fairly well predictable at the macro, 'social group' level at which most positivist sociology is done, for example, in predicting voting behaviour.

But many of the questions relevant to nursing practice are precisely at the micro level of the individual where the positivist scientific research model is of little help. The knowledge that woundcare method X is most appropriate for wounds of type A

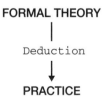

Figure 2.1 The scientific model of the relationship between theory and practice

tells us only that, *in the majority of cases in which it was tested*, it was found to be the most effective treatment. It tells us nothing about its effect on a particular patient P. This was referred to in Chapter 1 as the problem of deduction.

When a physicist says that paint X is the most effective paint for covering metal A, he means that in *all* cases of metal A under the same conditions, paint X will be the best paint to use. In contrast, when a nurse–researcher says that treatment X is the most effective treatment for healing wound type A, she usually means that in a statistically significant number of cases from a sample of patients with wound type A, treatment X was found to be the most effective. The research-based painter *knows* that paint X will be the most effective paint for covering his piece of metal, whereas the research-based nurse only *hopes* that treatment X will be the most effective treatment for this particular wound on this particular patient. Clearly, if we wish our research to have any direct impact on the care of patient X, then patient X must *participate* in that research, either as a subject or in some other way.

If the positivist social science model of research is unsuitable for generating knowledge about specific nurse–patient interactions, perhaps the interpretive, anti-positivist model will be of more use. This model was developed as a reaction to the positivists, whose founding fathers wished to construct 'a positive science of society' based on 'invariable laws' (Comte, 1976) in which 'collective ways of acting or thinking have a reality outside the individual' (Durkheim, 1938). The anti-positivists saw the social sciences as being concerned with something more than direct, rational understanding. Hence, Weber (1947) wrote of going *beyond* scientific understanding to 'accomplish something which is never attainable in the natural sciences, namely the subjective understanding of the action of the component individuals'.

Weber sought to distinguish between *Erklären* (explanation) and *Verstehen* (understanding), and claimed that whereas the aim of the natural sciences is merely to explain, the aim of the social sciences should be to understand at a deeper level. Furthermore, for Weber, this understanding could only be subjective, so the supposedly objective methods of science must of necessity be rejected. Thus, while Durkheim advised that 'the first and most fundamental rule is: consider social facts as things', Harré and Secord (1972) countered with 'for scientific purposes, treat people as if they were human beings'.

The interpretive model of social research would certainly appear to be more appropriate to our needs than positivism, emphasising as it does the reality of the individual social interaction and its emphasis on understanding rather than on explaining. However, although some of the anti-positivist methods and methodologies might well be of use in nursing, the adoption of the model in its entirety poses problems for the new paradigm nurse-researcher, since the aims of the interpretive model of social research are still concerned with the generation of knowledge. In contrast, it will be recalled that the nurse-practitioner bases her nursing practice on praxis, the coming together of theory and practice as the two sides of the same coin, and is concerned primarily with the development of practice.

Praxis implies that theory and practice cannot be separated, and that theory is generated out of practice, and informs new practice through the process of hypothesising. The relationship between theory and practice is not hierarchical, but mutually enhancing, and it makes no sense to talk either of theory *explaining* practice, as the positivists attempt to explain social reality, or of theory *understanding* practice as the anti-positivists attempt to understand social reality. If the theory-practice gap is to be dissolved, the aim of research for the nurse-practitioner should be directly to influence and bring about *change* in practice without the intervention of theory, in a way that the majority of social science methodologies are neither designed nor intended to do. As Carr and Kemmis (1986) pointed out, the problems of practical disciplines 'are always practical problems which, unlike theoretical problems, cannot be resolved by the discovery of new knowledge, but only by adopting some course of action'.

Towards a new model of nursing research

On first sight, it might not be thought possible to imagine a model of nursing research which bypasses theory and addresses nursing practice directly, particularly as nurses are currently being encouraged to adopt the model of research-based practice, in which research generates theory and theory directs practice in a linear, causal, hierarchical process. However, by distinguishing, as we did with the model of nursing praxis in the previous chapter, between formal macro theory and informal micro theory, the linear process becomes cyclical, and formal, research-based theory is reduced to informing rather than directing practice.

Positivist scientific research is still required to generate formal theory, but its role in shaping nursing praxis is secondary. What is now of greater importance is a model of research that will uncover and make sense of informal theory, theory that is generated directly out of practice, and that can only be achieved through establishing a direct relationship between research and practice, a relationship that is not mediated by formal, generalisable theory. We need a model of research which will formalise the process of reflective practice and elevate the status of informal, tacit, 'intuitive' knowledge and theory to the same or greater level as formal, research-based knowledge. It is only in this way that Benner's notion of the expert practitioner, with a vast wealth of past paradigm cases based on her own unique experience, will be realised.

What is required from a model of research for nursing praxis is therefore:

- that it will contribute towards the reduction of the theory–practice gap and the separation of practitioner from theorist by developing methodologies which can be applied by nurse–practitioners in their own clinical settings;
- that it will *directly* bring about improvements in nursing practice rather than merely contributing to generalisable knowledge and theory;
- that when it does address knowledge and theory, it will do so on an individual, micro level, contributing to an understanding of individual nurse–patient interactions.

It can be seen that such a model would oppose many of the principles currently taken for granted by researchers operating from within the technical rationality tradition. Much of the research generated by this new model would be small-scale project work, undertaken at a local level and not generalisable beyond the practice area in which it was conducted. It would be carried out by practitioners themselves, and perhaps even by patients, rather than by academics, and would often involve initiating changes in practice as an integral part of the research process. Indeed, a great deal of what would take place would probably not currently be recognised as research at all.

There are two ways in which the requirements of research for praxis can be realised. Firstly, the process of reflection-on-action can be refined into a model of *reflective* research whereby the nurse–practitioner generates personal knowledge and informal micro theory through reflection on her own practice. The knowledge and theory constructed in this way will not be generalisable beyond the kinds of situations and patients it was generated from, and therefore eliminates many of the problems of induction, verification and deduction, and dissolves the theory–practice gap.

Secondly, the traditional scientific research process can be extended to encompass the implementation of findings in a model of *reflexive* research. Just as reflective research dissolves the theory–practice gap by removing the necessity for generalisation, so reflexive research dissolves the gap by ensuring that clinical change occurs as part of the process of doing research. Reflective research contributes to nursing praxis by generating personal knowledge and informal theory which is then employed to construct and test hypotheses in the clinical situation; reflexive research contributes to nursing praxis, the coming together of theory and practice, by directly influencing practice. The implementation of clinical change in reflexive research is, by definition, as much a part of the research process as the generation of data: to do reflexive research is of necessity to impact upon the situation that you are researching. The process of reflexive research will be discussed in detail later in the chapter.

A hierarchy of nursing research

In the social sciences, from which the current dominant paradigm of nursing research was developed, the purpose of research is seen as the generation of formal, generalisable theory,

LEVEL 4	Implementation of Change
LEVEL 3	Individual, Micro Understanding
LEVEL 2	Global, Macro Understanding
LEVEL 1	Explanation

Figure 2.2 A nursing research hierarchy

with the main point of contention centring around the qualita-tive–quantitative debate, and whether social science should seek to understand or merely to explain. In nursing, however, there are the other perspectives outlined above: research should also be concerned with generating informal, micro theory and with changing and improving nursing practice. These separate and diverse aims of research can be organised into a hierarchy (Figure 2.2), with explanation at the bottom (Level 1), followed by macro, global understanding (Level 2), micro, individual understanding (Level 3), and with the direct implementation of change at the top (Level 4).

By categorising research in terms of its aims or purpose, the subjectivity–objectivity debate is also resolved, since no matter how carefully the researcher tries to avoid bias in the *collection* of data, raw data are of little use; they require analysis and inter-pretation in order to extract meaning from them. And since, as Lukes (1981) pointed out, there are many possible interpreta-tions that can be placed on any findings, subjectivity is inevitable if the data are to be of any practical use. Quantitative research findings might, on the surface, appear to be the result of an objective process, but that objectivity vanishes as soon as a theorist or practitioner attempts to apply them in the real world. The question is therefore not whether social and nursing research is subjective or objective, but at what point, and by whom, a subjective interpretation is introduced.

From this perspective, it can be seen that positivist and inter-pretive methodologies, being concerned with explanation (Level 1) and understanding (Level 2), respectively, simply repre-sent two stages in the transition from raw data to usable research findings. Level 1 research presents raw or almost raw data, data that might have been processed but would not have been analysed. The analysis of data from Level 1 studies is left to the reader or commissioning body of the research. Level 2 research might well present raw data, perhaps in the form of interview transcripts, but it will also provide the reader with an analysis of how those data contribute to an understanding of the phenomenon being studied.

Research at Levels 1 and 2 therefore corresponds very loosely to the quantitative and qualitative schools of social research, although the distinction is made according to the aims of the research rather than the methods employed. For that reason, there is often an overlap, with quantitative methods being employed in Level 2 research and, very occasionally, with qualitative methods being employed in Level 1 research.

Research at Levels 1 and 2 also maintains the gap between theory and practice, since as we have seen, the process of turning generalisable research findings into micro theory of relevance to individual nurse–practitioners with individual patients is flawed as a result of the problem of deduction. However, at Level 3, which is concerned with the generation of personal knowledge and informal, micro theory, and at Level 4, where clinical change comes about as a direct result of carrying out the research, no such problems occur. Therefore, whereas research at Levels 1 and 2 conforms to the traditional scientific paradigm, and generates formal theory for traditional research-based practice, Level 3 and 4 research is of far greater interest to the nurse–practitioner. Both types are required by nursing, but a glance through any journal will show that Level 3 and 4 research studies are few and far between, at least in the published literature.

Level 1 and 2 research

The purpose of Level 1 research is, as far as possible, to present objective findings in a neutral and unbiased fashion. Common methods are questionnaires and non-participant observation, as these are usually considered to possess high degrees of objectivity. Level 1 research reports might include short discussion and recommendation sections, but the emphasis will be on the presentation of the results. The Census is a good example of Level 1 research, since its function is to present a wide range of statistical data in neutral form to be interpreted by policy makers and social scientists for the purpose of analysis and social planning. An example from nursing might be a survey of patient satisfaction with care on a particular ward, the results of which would be interpreted and possibly acted upon by the hospital managers. Much audit work also falls into the category of Level 1 research due to its focus on objective, measurable outcomes.

Although the written report of a Level 1 study might attempt an analysis of the results and suggest certain recommendations, its remit ends with the presentation of the findings and it is the responsibility of someone other than the researcher to interpret and implement them. Therefore, many externally funded and commissioned projects are at Level 1, since commissioning bodies generally require neutral results which they can then interpret according to their particular needs and preconceptions, and recommend or implement action in line with their own policies.

Level 2 research continues the process to its next stage, and is primarily concerned with meaning and interpretation. Some surveys and questionnaires are at this level, but the majority of Level 2 studies employ a broadly phenomenological methodology, which 'advocates an approach to examining the empirical social world which requires the researcher to interpret the real world from the perspective of the subjects of his investigation' (Filstead, 1970). Whereas Level 1 researchers are asking questions such as 'what?' and 'how many?', Level 2 researchers are asking 'why?' and 'how come?'. They are not prepared to leave these questions to others, believing that the people in the best position to provide the answers are not outside agencies but the researchers and subjects themselves. Furthermore, whereas Level 1 studies produce *information* of use to planners and analysts, Level 2 research integrates that information into a theoretical framework to produce generalisable *knowledge*.

Typical methods employed in Level 2 research are semi-structured and unstructured interviews, which allow the subjects the opportunity to express their own thoughts and feelings in depth and in their own words; and participant observation, in which the researchers join the group they are investigating in order to experience for themselves the reality of being a group member.

There are many well-known examples of Level 2 research in the social sciences, for example, Goffman's study of life inside a mental hospital in the 1950s. Goffman took a job as a ward orderly in order to experience institutional life from the inside, and there is little doubt from reading the book of his experiences (Goffman, 1968) that it presents a very different picture than would the results of a questionnaire, or even the findings from a non-participant observation study. Nursing literature is littered with examples of Level 2 research: many quantitative studies and virtually all qualitative studies are concerned with interpreting and extracting meaning from the data.

Level 3 research

Level 3 research is based on the process of reflection-on-action, which in nursing is not usually perceived as a research method at all, but rather as a means of learning through experience or of improving practice. However, Fitzgerald offered the following definition of reflection-on-action as:

> the retrospective contemplation of practice undertaken in order to uncover the knowledge used in a particular situation, by analysing and interpreting the information recalled. The reflective practitioner may speculate how the situation might have been handled differently and what other knowledge would have been helpful. (Fitzgerald, 1994)

This view of reflection-on-action satisfies most of the definitions of nursing research found in Table 2.1 at the start of this chapter, by being planned and systematic, by leading to an increase in knowledge, albeit tacit, personal knowledge, and by identifying and developing (informal) theory. Where it falls down in traditional research terms is in not producing generalisable findings, that is, findings which can be applied to settings other than the one in which they were uncovered. However, it is ideally suited to nursing praxis where the main concern is the unique and individual relationship between patient and nurse.

Level 3 or reflective research is concerned primarily with researching one's own practice. It is an individual endeavour whose aim is to generate personal knowledge and informal theory from a retrospective, systematic and detailed analysis of what happened in the practice setting. It is a formal process of turning experience into knowledge and is a major contributory factor to what Benner (1984) referred to as expertise. It ideally suits the purpose of the nurse–practitioner, who is concerned with the integration of theory and practice through nursing praxis, since it enables her to generate knowledge and theory of direct relevance to her own individual therapeutic relationships with her patients. Reflective research therefore eliminates the theory–practice gap by ensuring that theory developed out of clinical encounters with a particular patient is directly applied back into the nurse's practice with that same patient.

Reflection-on-action can take many forms. It can be achieved through keeping a reflective diary or journal, through reflective conversations with critical friends, through debriefing, through clinical supervision, or through critical incident analysis. In order for it to constitute reflective research, however, it must be formally recorded, and where possible, publicly disseminated. It should be systematic and open to scrutiny and critique, and it is only by making public the process of reflection-on-action that we can hope to have it recognised as a bona fide research method, and the practice and theory resulting from it as legitimate.

If we wish to justify clinical decisions made on the basis of reflection-on-action, we must be able to produce written evidence of a systematic process of knowledge and theory generation. The purpose of making the reflective process available to others is therefore not, as with traditional positivist research, because it is generalisable and of direct use to other practitioners, since most reflection is clearly not, but because if we are to base our practice on our reflection-on-action, we must be able to openly demonstrate the source of our clinical decisions.

For the informal theory generated through the process of reflection-on-action to be of any practical use, it must be translated into nursing practice. It can be seen by returning to the model of nursing praxis (Figure 1.5) that the personal knowledge and paradigm cases resulting from reflection-on-action are used to construct informal theory in just the same way that empirical research findings are used to construct formal theory, and that both are then employed by the nurse–practitioner to inform and direct her practice through the process of hypothesising. However, there are two major differences in this model between formal and informal theory. Firstly, informal theory has a greater influence on practice than formal theory; and secondly, informal theory is generated by the nurse–practitioner herself rather than by an external researcher.

Reflection-on-action is therefore an important and valid form of research, carried out by the practitioner herself to inform her own practice, and one which completely removes the barriers between the researcher and the practitioner. Research, in the form of reflection-on-action applied to informal theory and hypothesis generation, becomes part of the everyday activity of the nurse–practitioner. She is constantly reflecting on her past and current practice, theorising and hypothesising from her reflections and modifying her nursing interventions accordingly. The researcher therefore retains complete control over how the findings from her work are implemented; indeed, it is impossible to separate the implementation from the research itself.

Level 4 research

Although Level 3 reflective research often results in improvements to practice, its primary aim is to generate informal theory. Level 4 research, on the other hand, is research for change; research with the implementation of change implicitly built-in. It is referred to in this book as reflexive research, since it is research which not only brings about change in practice, but is itself capable of being modified by that change, and in turn directs and modifies the change it is investigating in a continuous feedback loop. It is in many ways similar to the concept of theoretical sampling in grounded theory methodology (Glaser and Strauss, 1967), but is directed at generating new practice rather than new theory. We might therefore also refer to Level 4 reflexive research as grounded practice research.

The aim of reflexive research in nursing is not, as with Level 2 research, to generate formal theory, since as we have seen, the generation of formal theory does not very often result in clinical change. Neither is it, as with Level 3 research, to generate informal theory, although this might sometimes be produced as a by-product of carrying out the research. The difference between traditional Level 1 and 2 scientific research and reflexive research is therefore in its aims and purpose rather than its methods. And unlike Level 3 reflective research, which employs a methodology from outside the mainstream scientific paradigm, reflexive research often borrows its methods from the social sciences, albeit to a different end.

The purpose of Level 4 research is therefore not just to describe or explain, but to bring about change. It could, of course, be argued that all research aims to bring about change, but the decision to implement research findings, and the direction that the implementation takes, is usually in the hands of outside agencies. Thus, the Census does not in itself produce policy change, nor did Goffman's study result in direct improvements in psychiatric hospitals, although other people might use his findings to argue for reforms. But as Sayer (1992) pointed out, 'it is easy for the researchers to forget that changing people's thinking may leave the world of practice largely unchanged', and many published Level 1 and 2 research reports are simply not read and acted upon by the people with the power to implement their findings. And even when there is a will to act, we have seen that generalisable research findings do not readily translate into effective nursing practice on a micro level.

The difference between Level 1 and 2 research on the one hand, and Level 3 and 4 research on the other, is that Level 3 and 4 researchers retain control and direction over the implementation of their findings, and that the Level 4 research process *of itself* initiates and responds to change. What is more, Level 4 research transcends the quantitative–qualitative dichotomy that bedevils much nursing research, since any method can be employed to bring about change. The defining factor with regard to Level 4 research is not how it is carried out, but *why* it is carried out. In fact, it makes little sense to discuss research at this level in terms of methods at all; rather, we should speak of an approach to, a philosophy of, or attitude towards, research.

But Level 4 research is not about *any* change. It is concerned with bringing about positive therapeutic change in the patients that the nurse–practitioner is working with, and in order for reflexive research to say anything meaningful about an individual patient, that patient must somehow be involved in the research process. This involvement might be as a research subject in a small-scale, localised study, but reflexive research can also be carried out by patients, clients and carers, either in partnership with their practitioners, or independently.

Level 4 research as reflection-in-action

The simplest form of Level 4 research is reflection-in-action, since:

> When someone reflects-in-action, he becomes a researcher in the practice context. He is not dependant on the categories of established theory and techniques, but constructs a new theory of the unique case. His inquiry is not limited to a deliberation about means which depends on a prior agreement about ends. He does not keep means and ends separate, but defines them interactively as he frames a problematic situation. He does not separate thinking from doing, ratiocinating his way to a decision which he must later convert to action. Because his experimenting is a kind of action, implementation is built into his inquiry. (Schön, 1983)

This description clearly meets the criteria for Level 4 research, and therefore, as with reflective research, reflexive research is part of the everyday practice of the nurse–practitioner. But if we wish reflection-in-action to be recognised as a formal research method as well as a way of doing nursing practice, then it must be located within a methodological framework.

Fortunately, we already have just such a framework in the model of nursing praxis shown in Figure 1.5. It will be recalled that nursing praxis becomes reflection-in-action or on-the-spot experimenting when the nurse–practitioner is able to continue round the cycle without the need to engage in reflection-on-action away from the clinical area; in other words, when reflection-on-action becomes something that can be carried out on the spot during practice. The nurse–practitioner is therefore not only constructing informal micro theory, but is actively testing out that theory by implementing it with her patient, and reflexively modifying it as a result of her interventions. This form of Level 4 research is based on the scientific method of hypothetico-abductivism, and therefore lies outside of the formal scientific paradigm, but there are a number of more traditional ways that Level 4 research can be conducted.

Level 4 research as single case research

One possible model for Level 4 research is the single case methodology which derives from applied behavioural analysis in psychology, since clients from the practitioner's own clinical work are used as research subjects. The most basic form of single case research is the simple time series or A-B design, in which baseline measurements are taken (A), an intervention is introduced, and further measurements are taken (B) to determine the effectiveness of that intervention. Morley (1989) pointed out that causal relationships are difficult to attribute from a simple A-B design, and so an A-B-A-B design, in which treatment is repeatedly withdrawn and reintroduced, is often employed.

Although this model satisfies the criterion for Level 4 research that change should be implicitly built-in to the research process, there are two problems with adopting single case research as a reflexive, Level 4 approach. The first is concerned with the ethics of repeatedly introducing and withdrawing a nursing intervention, and the second is concerned with the nature of the resulting therapeutic change: there is no guarantee that the change introduced in single case research will be beneficial to patients. If it proves not to be, of course, it will be withdrawn, but then the research intervention will not have fulfilled the Level 4 criterion of bringing about change. Furthermore, since the treatment at each stage has to be the same, this model is not truly reflexive, as the implementation of change is not immediately responsive to the emerging findings.

These problems can be resolved by converting the linear A-B design into a cyclical feedback loop, in which a baseline measure is taken, an intervention is introduced, its effect is measured, further changes are introduced, the effects of which are in turn measured, and so on, until the desired positive therapeutic change is achieved. Any methods can be employed to measure the therapeutic change, which can be continually modified, and thus a positive outcome is guaranteed by the cyclical nature and reflexivity of the research design.

Level 4 research as action research

This modified single case approach might seem on first sight to be very similar to the social science model of action research, which was developed by Kurt Lewin (1947) from wartime operational research. Action research is problem-centred, and is based on a cycle of theory generation, testing, evaluation and modification. This could be seen as a useful model for Level 4 research, since change is very clearly built into the action research process, and is an inevitable consequence of carrying out the research. Applied to nursing, it offers the promise of bringing about positive change in the health of patients (Greenwood, 1994) and of closing the theory-practice gap (Webb, 1990). However, as with single case research, there are several problems with this model as it stands if it is to be employed by the nurse-practitioner as part of the activity of nursing praxis.

Firstly, although action research, by its very title, promises change, as with all social science research it is grounded in theory generation rather than practice development. The purpose of implementing change in classic action research was generally not primarily for the sake of bringing about improvements in the situation under investigation, but rather to test theories empirically, to discover whether they worked when applied in the real world. Therefore, although action research often resulted in change, the change was secondary to the development of theory, and was not always change for the better.

Secondly, action researchers were generally commissioned by an organisation rather than being part of it. There is no concept in the traditional model of action research of practitioners researching their own practice, but rather of scientists coming in and implementing change based on a theoretical framework in order to determine whether the theory 'fits' the real life situation. This model neither reduces the theory-practice gap, since practice is still determined by theory, nor does it bring the theoretician and practitioner closer together, since the distinction between them is not only maintained but reinforced by the theorist encroaching physically into the practitioner's territory.

Thirdly, traditional action research attempted to maintain objectivity and to work within the formal scientific paradigm. Action research was generally undertaken on behalf of a client, and the action researcher attempted to promote the image of an impartial scientist coming in to test theories in real-life situations to see whether the predictions made from them were borne out in practice. The role of the researcher was therefore to 'serve as professional expert, designing the project, gathering the data, interpreting the findings and recommending action to the client organization. Like the conventional model of pure research, this is an elitist model of research relationships' (Whyte, 1991). In short, the traditional version of action research is simply an extension of the technical rationality model in which the researcher not only proposes theories for the technician to implement in the practice situation, but actually comes into the practice area to *ensure* that they are implemented.

Usher and Bryant observed that these traditional views of action research:

> are limited by virtue of the fact that they do not consider the possibilities of practitioners doing their own research. The net result of their particular orientations is to 'save' action research for positivism and foundationalism through maintaining a separate domain of academic research expertise and preserving those theory–practice distinctions.... (Usher and Bryant, 1989)

The discipline of education has responded by developing a new model of action research which addresses those criticisms. Elliott (1991) has defined action research simply as 'the study of a social situation with a view to improving the quality of action within it', and this, as Altrichter *et al.* have pointed out:

> directs attention to one of the most essential motives for doing action research. It lies in the will to improve the quality of teaching and learning as well as the conditions under which teachers and students work in schools. Action research is intended to support teachers, and groups of teachers, in coping with the challenges and problems of practice and carrying through innovations in a reflective way. Experience with action research, so far, has shown that teachers are able to do this successfully and can achieve remarkable results when given opportunities and support. (Altrichter *et al.*, 1993)

The discipline of education is clearly much further down the road of reflexive research than is nursing, and the interested reader is referred to the excellent book by Altrichter *et al.* (1993) for a step-by-step guide to carrying out action research in an educational setting which is readily transferable to nursing.

Ebbutt has produced a more comprehensive definition of action research in education as:

> The systematic study of attempts to change and improve educational
> practice by groups of participants by means of their own practical
> actions and by means of their own reflection upon the effects of those
> actions. (Ebbutt, 1985)

We need only substitute the word 'educational' with 'nursing' to
make it relevant to this discussion. Usher and Bryant (1989)
pointed out that this definition makes four claims about the
nature of action research. It is research which:

- is carried out by practitioners, or at least, that researchers are
  actually participating in the practices being researched, and
  working collaboratively with practitioners;
- improves practice through transformation of the practice
  situation. In the words of Schön (1983) 'the practitioner has
  an interest in transforming the situation from what it is to
  something he likes better';
- involves a process of reflection on, and understanding of,
  action and its outcomes, and of acting through understanding;
- is systematic in its approach, and is open to public scrutiny
  and critique.

It can be seen that this approach to doing research is necessarily
subjective in that the changes it attempts to bring about are
changes which are considered desirable by the researcher.
Furthermore, it breaks down the division between researcher
and practitioner by encouraging the nurse to research her own
practice and to modify practice as a result of that research.

The issue of subjectivity is of particular relevance to the Level
4 researcher, and is implicit in the concept of reflexivity. It was
stated earlier that reflexive research is based on the feedback
loop, that the findings from the research modify the practice
situation being studied, which alters the findings, which
modifies practice, and so on. In this way, practice is being continuously shaped by the process of doing the research, but it is
important that it is being changed *for the better*, and this entails
a series of subjective, qualitative decisions by the researchers as
to what constitutes improvements in practice. In the words of
Schön quoted earlier, the researcher 'has an interest in transforming the situation from what it is to something he likes
better'. Level 4 reflexive research is therefore unashamedly

subjective in that it is the researchers themselves who are trans-lating their findings into practice, and where this differs from traditional scientific research is that it is happening in real time as part of the research process, and is thus far more explicit.

Usher and Bryant observed that this model of action research has itself been criticised by the positivist, technical rationality school of social science as lying outside the traditional scientific paradigm, as lacking in objectivity, and as not being generalis-able. However, from the perspective of the nurse–practitioner, these are the very qualities which make the model ideal for researching nursing praxis on a micro, interpersonal level. Returning to the requirements of a model of research for nursing praxis outlined earlier in the chapter, this new model of action research contributes towards the reduction of the theory-practice gap by enabling nurse–practitioners to research their own practice; it directly brings about improvements in nursing practice by having positive change built-in to the research process; and it generates informal, micro theory by focusing on the practitioner's individual nurse–patient interactions.

Level 4 research as co-operative inquiry

Although this model of action research integrates the roles of practitioner and researcher, reflexive research must also consider the role of the patient in the research process if it is to respond to the needs of the nurse–practitioner for micro theory about individual nurse–patient interactions. This issue was first addressed by co-operative or new paradigm research in the late 1970s and early 1980s (Reason and Rowan, 1981). Co-operative inquiry saw research as being with or for people rather than on them, and has been described as:

> a way of doing research in which all those involved contribute both to the creative thinking that goes into the enterprise — deciding on what is to be looked at, the methods of the inquiry, and making sense of what is found out — and also contribute to the action which is the subject of the research. (Reason, 1988)

Whereas action research and reflective research break down the distinction between researcher and practitioner, co-operative inquiry goes one step further and advocates that researcher, practitioner and research subject be seen as equal partners, each with a say in what is to be researched, how it will be done, and how the findings will be presented and implemented. It often involves the use of co-operative inquiry groups, in which each participant carries out research on themselves and on all the other members of the group.

Co-operative inquiry is of particular interest to the Level 4 researcher because of its philosophy of ownership of research findings by those involved in carrying out the research, and its emphasis on active participation in the implementation of those findings. Hence:

> Co-operative inquiry seeks knowledge in action and for action. Co-operative researchers may write books and articles, but often the knowledge that is really important for them is the practical knowledge of new skills and abilities.... And thus in co-operative inquiry, education and social action may become fully integrated with the research process. (Reason, 1988)

Several recent attempts have been made to combine action research and co-operative inquiry into a new model of research.

Hart and Bond (1995) have constructed a typology of action research for health and social care consisting of four categories, namely experimental, organisational, professionalising and empowering. Of these, the former two categories are similar to the traditional approaches to action research described earlier, and do not qualify as Level 4 research, while the latter two categories more closely resemble the model of action research being advocated in this book. More precisely, the professionalising type is similar to Usher and Bryant's description of reflexive action research, while the empowering type is similar to co-operative inquiry as described by Reason and Rowan.

Carr and Kemmis (1986) suggested three types of action research based on Habermas's three 'knowledge–constitutive interests' which he labelled the technical, the practical and the emancipatory (Habermas, 1972). Thus, 'technical action research occurs when facilitators persuade practitioners to test the findings of external research in their own practices'. In practical action research:

outside facilitators form co-operative relationships with practitioners, helping them to articulate their own concerns, plan strategic action for change, monitor the problems and effects of changes, and reflect on the value and consequences of the changes actually achieved. (Carr and Kemmis, 1986)

And in emancipatory action research, 'the practitioner group takes joint responsibility for the development of practice, understandings and situations', and the role of the outside researcher is minimal to the extent that 'an outsider taking such a role [of facilitator] would actually undermine the group's collaborative responsibility for the process' (Carr and Kemmis, 1986). Thus, of the three approaches, only emancipatory action research could accurately be described as a Level 4 approach, although practical action research comes close, particularly if it is designed reflexively.

In nursing, Holter and Schwartz-Barcott (1993) have identified three types of action research which clearly mirror those of Carr and Kemmis: the technical collaborative approach which aims to 'test a particular intervention based on a pre-specified theoretical framework'; the mutual collaborative approach, which 'brings researcher and practitioner together to identify problems and seek out possible causes and ways of intervening to change them'; and the enhancement approach which seeks to 'assist practitioners in identifying and making explicit fundamental problems by first raising their collaborative consciousness'.

Hart and Bond compared these three approaches to their own experimental, organisational and professionalising types of action research, but noted that there is no nursing equivalent to the empowering type of action research in which practitioner and patient work together. Furthermore, Holter and Schwartz-Barcott carried out a survey of the nursing literature and concluded that:

while the majority of the studies reported in nursing using action research can be placed under the technical collaborative approach to action research and a few studies can be placed as inquiries within the mutual collaborative approach, no studies have been found which convey the enhancement approach to action research. (Holter and Schwartz-Barcott, 1993)

What is required for Level 4 nursing research is therefore a greater emphasis on Hart and Bond's professionalising type action research, in which practitioners identify, carry out and implement findings from research in their own clinical areas, together with a new model similar to their empowering type action research, which brings together the nurse–practitioner and her patients in generating personal knowledge and informal theory of direct relevance to individual therapeutic relationships.

Together, these two approaches to Level 4 research will go some way towards diminishing the power of the external scientist-researcher; moving away from the old, outdated model of the nurse–technician; generating direct and immediate change in nursing practice as a result of practitioner *and* patient involvement at every stage of the research process, including the implementation of findings; and thereby dissolving the present gulf between theories which cannot and do not work, and practice which has changed and developed beyond the constraints of the traditional scientific paradigm. Several examples of this approach to Level 4 research are given in Part 2 of the book.

Research methods at Level 4

The reader will be aware that we have talked a great deal about a philosophy or methodology of Level 4 research, but have not, as yet, mentioned any specific methods. The reason for this is that Level 4 research is more concerned with ends than with means. It is concerned with generating informal theory, but more importantly, with bringing about clinical change. In traditional social science research, means and ends are closely entwined. If the researcher believes that the aim of social science is to understand social processes at a deep and meaningful level, then she must employ methods that will uncover meaning, such as phenomenology or ethnography.

In nursing praxis, however, where the aim of research is to integrate theory and practice into a seamless whole by generating practice and theory simultaneously, the methods are very much secondary to the aim of improving nursing practice. It is the philosophy of action through co-operation and integration that is important, and any methods are permissible so long as the impetus for reflexive change is built-in, either through practitioner involvement, patient involvement, or both.

An example will be taken from my own practice of teaching, which is expanded upon in Part 2 of this book and elsewhere (Jasper, 1994; Rolfe, 1994). A colleague and I wished to evaluate a course that we had co-written and jointly taught. Rather than employ traditional evaluation tools, in which the power and control over the process is retained by the teachers who are evaluating their own practice and who are free to disregard any findings that they find threatening or disagreeable, we attempted to employ a Level 4 research approach using co-operative inquiry.

This entailed providing the students with the time, space and resources to plan and carry out their own course evaluation and for them to submit a report of findings and recommendations, which we made a commitment to implement. The students identified for themselves the issues that they wanted to research and evaluate and the methods by which data would be collected. They maintained complete control over the interpretation and presentation of that data, and worked with us on its implementation into the course.

The students employed a wide range of different data collection methods, including questionnaires, attitude scales and interviews, and while some of the methods were, from a positivist scientific perspective, flawed and biased, these flaws and biases were employed creatively in discussions to probe the underlying motivations for asking particular research questions in particular ways. The end result was a collection of very rich findings which could never have been produced using traditional research methods, and which were owned by the students, who ensured their implementation.

Before moving on, however, it is important to note several objections to such an approach to research in nursing. Firstly, Greenwood (1994) has pointed out that the action research 'classics' were all written by teacher educators rather than by nurses, and that:

> Teachers enjoy autonomy in their classrooms which enables them, without risk, to implement small-scale innovation and even their truly emancipatory actions affects relatively few power brokers. The same is not true for clinical nurses. Nurses do not enjoy any real autonomy in multidisciplinary hospital practice, which means that even small-scale innovation has an impact on other more powerful health care professionals or managers. The effects of truly emancipatory action by nurses could, therefore, be profound.

Of course, a profound effect is precisely what we are hoping for, but this is nevertheless a very apposite point. To some extent, we are caught in a paradox in which the kind of paradigm shift being advocated in this book, where nurses will be recognised as researchers in their own right, will only come about as a *result* of nurses taking on this extended role. The solution is probably to start small with projects that will have a direct impact on our own practice, but which will not create too many ripples for the wider multidisciplinary team, and gradually extend outwards.

This leads to the second objection that action research is only appropriate for small-scale projects on wards or small units, but becomes problematic with larger populations (Sparrow and Robinson, 1994). This might well be true, but Level 4 research is, by definition, small scale since it seeks to involve researchers and research subjects as equal partners in bringing about local change of direct benefit to themselves.

And thirdly, if the aim of research is to improve practice for the benefit of service users and to involve those users as far as possible in the process of change, then we must recognise that:

> there may be competing definitions of what counts as improvement and success, and this may include differences between professionals and users of the service and/or between different professional groups.
> (Smith and Cantley, 1985)

This is an important point which deserves serious consideration. In theory, it should not present a problem, since, by definition, practitioners and service users will collaborate in the research as equal partners with an equal say in the direction that the research takes. However, the reality is that the power differential is very difficult to overcome, and there is a constant danger that the more powerful groups will take over the process and impose their own agenda. All that can be said is that as nurses or educationalists, we should be constantly aware of our potential for dominating the research agenda, and work to ensure that an equal, mutually empowering relationship between nurses and patients or educators and students develops with time.

A model of research for the nurse–practitioner

It has been argued in this chapter that the existence of the theory-practice gap in nursing is due in large part to the problem of deduction, of attempting to apply generalisable, Level 1 and 2 research findings generated through the scientific, technical rationality paradigm, to the work of the nurse-practitioner who is concerned more and more with unique and individual interactions between a single nurse and a single patient. Two ways in which research can address the clinical needs of the nurse-practitioner have been discussed: firstly, through reflective or Level 3 research; and secondly, through reflexive or Level 4 research. The four levels of the nursing research hierarchy are summarised in Table 2.2.

The example of nursing responses to patients who have attempted suicide will be used to illustrate the differences between research at the four levels. A Level 1 study into suicide might ask the question: '*What* are the social and demographic factors associated with suicide attempts?', with the aim of *explaining* the relationship between attempted suicide and variables such as social class, age and gender. In order to answer such a question, a *quantitative* approach would probably be

Table 2.2 A new model of nursing research

	Level 1	*Level 2*	*Level 3*	*Level 4*
Methodology	Positivist	Interpretive	Reflective	Reflexive
Function	Explanation	Macro understanding	Micro understanding	Change
Research questions	What?	Why? (generally)	Why? (specifically)	How?
Methods	Usually quantitative	Usually qualitative	Reflection-on-action	Reflection-in-action or any
Outcome of research	Information	Generalisable knowledge and formal theory	Personal knowledge and informal theory	Action
Relationship of research to nursing	Nursing is informed by research	Nursing is based on research	Nursing is integrated with research	Nursing is driven by research

taken, perhaps administering questionnaires to patients, or through statistical analysis of hospital records. The aim of the study would be to present statistical data showing correlations between variables in as objective a way as possible, thereby providing *information* for use in planning nursing services, and contributing to the development of nursing as a *research-informed* profession.

A Level 2 study into suicide might ask: '*Why* do people in general attempt suicide?', with the aim of *understanding* patients' reasons and motives. It is likely that a *qualitative* approach would be employed, possibly using semi-structured or depth interviews with patients who had made attempts on their own lives. The aim of the study would be to encourage the subjects to interpret and analyse their stated reasons for attempting suicide, extending existing *knowledge* in this field, and contributing to the development of nursing as a *research-based* profession.

A Level 3 study into suicide might ask: '*Why* do the patients I work with commit suicide, and what can I, *through my own practice*, do about it?', using the method of *reflection-on-action*. The nurse would reflect on her work with patients who had made suicide attempts, perhaps using critical incident analysis to examine good and bad examples from her own practice. New informal theories about working with people who had attempted suicide could be formulated, and new approaches to working with these patients could be tried out in clinical situations, their effectiveness reflected upon, and modifications made accordingly. In this way, the nurse would construct *informal theory* and 'a situational repertoire which is forever being expanded and modified to meet new situations' (Schön, 1983), developing expertise and 'a deep background understanding of clinical situations based on many past paradigm cases' (Benner, 1984), thereby *integrating* research into everyday practice.

A Level 4 study into suicide might ask: '*How* can the rate of attempted suicide be reduced?', with the aim of directly *changing* the number of presentations to the A&E Department. Either qualitative or quantitative methods could be employed, perhaps in an action research project in which staff introduced changes in their everyday clinical practice and monitored the outcomes over time, reflexively modifying the changes as necessary until the desired reductions in the suicide rate were achieved. The aim of the project would therefore be to promote nursing *action* and to contribute to nursing as a *research-driven* profession.

In one sense, this hierarchical model of nursing research represents a smooth transition of outcomes from the generation of information (Level 1) through to the direct implementation of change (Level 4). In another sense, however, there is a clear dichotomy between research at Levels 1 and 2 on the one hand, and research at Levels 3 and 4 on the other. Level 1 and 2 research:

- is located in the scientific, technical rationality paradigm;
- attempts to be objective and rigorous;
- aims to uncover generalisable information, knowledge and theory;
- is based on a technical model of nursing as caring for;
- sees a clear distinction between the researcher and practitioner and hence between theory and practice;
- supports research-based practice.

Level 3 and 4 research:

- circumvents the processes of induction, verification and deduction;
- is unashamedly subjective and often lacks formal, scientific rigour;
- aims to generate personal knowledge and theory as well as directly bringing about clinical change;
- is based on a humanistic model of nursing as caring *about*;
- sees no distinction between the researcher and practitioner (and sometimes the patient), who are usually the same person; and hence dissolves the gap between theory and practice;
- aims for the integration of practice and research, and supports research-driven practice.

Therefore, while Level 1 and 2 research remains a useful source of generalisable knowledge and theory to inform the nurse–practitioner in her work, its importance is diminished, to be replaced by Level 3 and 4 research which the nurse-practitioner carries out for herself as part of her everyday practice, and which provides personal, tacit knowledge and informal micro theory of relevance to the encounters between the nurse–practitioner and her individual patients, as well as having a direct impact on clinical practice.

Unfortunately, however, the nursing profession is moving ever closer to the traditional scientific paradigm and Level 1 and 2 research. The publication in 1993 of the Report of the *Taskforce on the Strategy for Research in Nursing, Midwifery and Health Visiting* (Department of Health, 1993) considered two options for nursing research: that it should be fully integrated into the wider body of healthcare research, currently dominated by the medical profession; or that it should be seen as a special case, different from research in other areas of healthcare. While it has been argued in this chapter that nursing research should be different from medical and other forms of healthcare research simply because nursing is different from medicine and other forms of healthcare, the Taskforce chose the other option, committing nursing research to the narrow, scientific, elitist path trodden by most medical research. The definition of research adopted by the Taskforce conforms precisely to the descriptions in this chapter of Level 1 and Level 2 research, and argues along the traditional scientific lines of knowledge generation, generalisability, rigour and elitism.

Elitism in nursing research is particularly damaging to the profession. The Taskforce emphasised the point that 'not... all practitioners should be carrying out research as part of their professional role or their professional development'; that 'much of the research undertaken [by nurses and midwives] is small-scale project-type work'; that 'a majority of the studies... are not externally funded and are carried out within the individuals' own time', thereby not qualifying as 'real' research; and that 'the proliferation of inadequately supervised, small-scale projects should be curbed' (Department of Health, 1993).

These statements are both worrying and encouraging: worrying in that an eminent body largely comprised of academics and managers has set an agenda for nursing research which is exerting a huge influence over the activities of nurse–researchers all over the country; but encouraging in that there is clearly enough 'small-scale project-type work' currently going on to worry the Taskforce into calling for it to be curbed. Adrian Webb, the Chair of the Taskforce, has expressed a wish that the Report should 'facilitate a debate within nursing, health visiting and midwifery — and more generally — rather than signal an end to the promising dialogues which we have been able to initiate with a variety of bodies' (Department of Health, 1993). It is important that ordinary practising nurses add their voices to this debate to point out the limitations of traditional scientific paradigm research to their work, and to express concern over its inability to bridge the theory–practice gap. It is only by listening to the needs and concerns of those nurses who require usable research findings to improve and develop their own practice, that nursing research will ever properly address the real requirements of the profession.

A vision for the future

This chapter will conclude by examining two visions of the researcher–practitioner, written over 370 years apart. The first is by Sir Francis Bacon, often hailed as the father of modern scientific method, who observed that:

> Those who have handled sciences have been either men of experiment or men of dogmas. The men of experiment are like the ant, they only collect and use: the reasoners resemble spiders, who make cobwebs out of their own substance. But the bee takes a middle course: it gathers its material from the flowers of the garden and of the field, but transforms and digests it by a power of its own. (Bacon, 1620)

The ants are the scientific researchers, who construct knowledge and theories out of empirical data, whereas the spiders are theoreticians, who formulate theories and models 'out of their own substance', that is, from within themselves. But the bees, the researcher–practitioners, not only gather their own data 'from the flowers of the garden and of the field', but transform those data into knowledge and theory 'by a power of its own'. They not only collect like the ant, but construct like the spider.

The second quotation comes from the discipline of education which, as we saw earlier, is much further down the road to reflexive research than is nursing. Altrichter *et al.* described the characteristics and achievements of teachers who have engaged in reflexive action research, and the full quotation will be reproduced here, but with all references to teaching changed to nursing in order to demonstrate where nursing could be in 10 years time if nurses are encouraged to develop and carry out reflective and reflexive research into their own practice.

> These [nurses] have not only carried out developmental work for their [clinical areas] but have also broadened their knowledge and their professional competency. They have passed on this knowledge to colleagues, [patients, carers] and, in written form, also to the wider public. They have shown that [nurses] can make an important contribution to the knowledge base of their profession. And they have demonstrated that they can engage successfully with professional problems without recourse to external direction. They did not restrict their work to adopting a set of practical routines, but acted as professionals precisely in developing new theories about their practice, including a critique of its [medical] and social contexts.
>
> These [nurses] are 'normal' [nurses], who reflect on their practice to strengthen and develop its positive features. They are not prepared to accept blindly the problems they face from day to day, but instead they reflect upon them and search for solutions and improvements. They are committed to building on their strengths and to overcoming their weaknesses. They wish to experiment with new ideas and strategies, rather than letting their practice petrify. (Altrichter *et al.*, 1993)

These researcher–practitioners are clearly bee men and women, transforming the pollen of research into the honey of practice, employing a seventeenth-century model for twenty-first-century nursing research.

References

Altrichter, H., Posch, P. and Somekh, B. (1993) *Teachers Investigate their Work*. London: Routledge.

Bacon, F. (1620) First book of aphorisms. Cited in M. Hollis *The Philosophy of Social Science*. Cambridge: Cambridge University Press.

Benner, P. (1984) *From Novice to Expert*. California: Addison-Wesley.

Bond, S. (1993) Experimental research in nursing: necessary but not sufficient. In: *Nursing: Art and Science* (A. Kitson, ed.) London: Chapman and Hall.

Burns, N. and Grove, S.K. (1987) *The Practice of Nursing Research*. Philadelphia: W.B. Saunders.

Carr, W. and Kemmis, S. (1986) *Becoming Critical.* London: Falmer Press.

Chapman, J. (1991) Research — what it is and what it is not. In: *Nursing: a Knowledge Base for Practice* (A. Perry and M. Jolley, eds). London: Edward Arnold.

Clark, J.M. and Hockey, L. (1989) *Further Research for Nursing.* London: Scutari.

Cohen, L. and Manion, L. (1985) *Research Methods in Education.* London: Croom Helm.

Comte, A. (1976) *The Foundations of Sociology.* London: Nelson.

Department of Health (1993) *Report of the Taskforce on the Strategy for Research in Nursing, Midwifery and Health Visiting.* London: DoH.

Durkheim, E. (1938) *The Rules of Sociological Method.* New York: The Free Press.

Ebbutt, D. (1985) Educational action research: some general concerns and specific quibbles. In: *Issues in Educational Research: Qualitative Methods* (R.G. Burgess, ed.) Lewes: Falmer Press.

Elliott, J. (1991) *Action Research for Educational Change.* Milton Keynes: Open University Press.

Elliott, J. and Ebbutt, D. (1985) *Issues in Teaching for Understanding.* Harlow: Longmans, for Schools Council.

Field, P.A. and Morse, J.M. (1985) *Nursing Research.* London: Chapman and Hall.

Filstead, W.J. (1970) *Qualitative Methodology.* Slough: Markham.

Fitzgerald, M. (1994) Theories of reflection for learning. In: *Reflective Practice in Nursing* (A. Palmer, S. Burns and C. Bulman, eds) Oxford: Blackwell Scientific.

Glaser, B.G. and Strauss, A.L. (1967) *The Discovery of Grounded Theory.* New York: Aldine.

Goffman, E. (1968) *Asylums.* Harmondsworth: Penguin.

Greenwood, J. (1994) Action research: a few details, a caution and something new. *J. Adv. Nursing,* **20**, 13–18.

Habermas, J. (1972) *Knowledge and Human Interests.* London: Heinemann.

Harré, R. (1979) *Social Being.* Oxford: Blackwell.

Harré, R. and Secord, P.F. (1972) *The Explanation of Social Behaviour.* Oxford: Blackwell.

Hart, E. and Bond, M. (1995) *Action Research for Health and Social Care.* Buckingham: Open University Press.

Heisenberg, W. (1963) *Physics and Philosophy.* London: Allen and Unwin.

Holter, I.M. and Schwartz-Barcott, D. (1993) Action research: what is it? How has it been used and how can it be used in nursing? *J. Adv.*

Nursing, **18**, 298-304.

Hunt, J. (1982) The recognition battle. *Nursing Mirror*, **154**(9), March 3, 24-26.

Jasper, M. (1994) A shortened common foundation programme for graduates — the students experience of student-centred learning. *Nurse Education Today*, **14**, 238-244.

Lancaster, A. (1975) Nursing, nurses and research. *Nursing Times*, **71**, May 15, 42-44.

Lewin, K. (1947) Frontiers in group dynamics: social planning and action research. *Hum. Relat.*, **1**(2), 143-153.

Lukes, S. (1981) Fact and theory in the social sciences. In: *Society and the Social Sciences* (D. Potter, ed.) London: Routledge and Kegan Paul.

MacGuire, J. (1991) Tailoring research for advanced nursing practice. In: *Nursing as Therapy* (R. McMahon and A. Pearson, eds) London: Chapman and Hall.

May, T. (1993) *Social Research*. Buckingham: Open University Press.

Morley, S. (1989) Single case research. In: *Behavioural and Mental Health Research* (G. Parry and F.N. Watts, eds) Hove: Lawrence Erlbaum Associates.

Reason, P. (1988) *Human Inquiry in Action*. London: Sage.

Reason, P. and Rowan, J. (1981) *Human Inquiry*. Chichester: Wiley.

Rolfe, G. (1994) Listening to students: course evaluation as action research. *Nurse Education Today*, **14**, 223-227.

Sarantakos, S (1994) *Social Research*. Basingstoke: Macmillan.

Sayer, A. (1992) *Method in Social Science*. London: Routledge.

Schön, D.A. (1983) *The Reflective Practitioner*. London: Temple Smith.

Smith, G. and Cantley, C. (1985) *Assessing Health Care: a Study in organizational Evaluation*. Milton Keynes: Open University Press.

Sparrow, S. and Robinson, J. (1994) Action research: an appropriate design for research in nursing? *Educational Action Research*, **2**(3), 347-355.

Treece, E.W. and Treece, J.W. (1986) *Elements of Research in Nursing*. St Louis: C.V. Mosby.

Usher, R. and Bryant, I. (1989) *Adult Education as Theory, Practice and Research*. London: Routledge.

Walker, R. (ed.) (1985) *Applied Qualitative Research*. Aldershot: Gower.

Webb, C. (1990) Partners in research. *Nursing Times*, **86**(32), 40-44.

Weber, M. (1947) The interpretive understanding of social action. In: *Readings in the Philosophy of the Social Sciences* (M. Brodbeck, ed.) (1968) New York: Macmillan.

Whyte, W.F. (1991) *Participatory Action Research*. New York: Sage.

3

Educating the nurse-practitioner

It seems to me that anything that can be taught to another is relatively inconsequential and has little or no significance on behaviour

Carl Rogers

Thank you Master for teaching me nothing

Old Zen story

Technocratic education and the nurse–technician

A hierarchy of theory and practice

In the previous chapters, a distinction was made between the nurse–technician, who operates within the technical rationality model of nursing and is concerned with the application of scientific, research-based theory to nursing practice, and the nurse–practitioner for whom the traditional scientific model has only limited relevance, and who is more concerned with generating her own theory from practice through reflection. It was also noted that the nursing profession continues to support the former model, despite a growing number of complaints from practitioners that it no longer meets the needs of current practice, which is ever more concerned with individualised patient care and one-to-one therapeutic relationships. These are issues which the traditional scientific model has difficulty in addressing, resulting in a gap between the theory and practice of nursing.

The commitment to a particular model of practice by a profession is probably best exemplified by the way in which it educates its future members. In nursing, the continued support given to the technical rationality model is clearly reflected in two educational developments which are currently exerting a profound influence on the profession: firstly, in the move of nurse education into the university sector; and secondly, in the structure and content of the Project 2000 curriculum.

From the dominant scientific perspective of nursing the move into higher education was timely, since, as Schön (1987) pointed out, most professional schools within modern universities are based on the technical rationality model in which 'practical competence becomes professional when its instrumental problem solving is grounded in systematic, preferably scientific knowledge'. Furthermore:

> As professional schools have sought to attain higher levels of academic rigor and status, they have oriented themselves towards an ideal most vividly represented by a particular view of medical education: physicians are thought to be trained as biotechnical problem solvers by immersion, first in medical science and then in supervised clinical practice where they learn to apply research-based techniques to diagnosis, treatment, and prevention. (Schön, 1987)

This model perfectly describes the aim of the Project 2000 curriculum, and suggests a hierarchy and sequencing of knowledge from basic science to applied science to technical skills of day-to-day practice. Furthermore, 'the greater one's proximity to basic science, as a rule, the higher one's academic status' (Schön, 1987). In the non-rigorous, 'minor professions' (Glazer, 1974) which arguably include nursing, 'yearning for the rigor of science-based knowledge and the power of science-based technique leads the schools to import scholars from neighbouring departments of social science' (Schön, 1987), and in the case of nursing, also from departments of psychology and life science. Academic credibility is therefore associated primarily with the hard sciences, and to a lesser extent with the softer social and behavioural sciences, and any deviations from the scientific paradigm are judged accordingly.

Bines (1992) supported the above analysis, and proposed three models of professional education, namely the pre-technocratic, the technocratic and the post-technocratic. Prior to the Project 2000 curriculum, nurse education adhered to the pre-technocratic model in which 'professional education takes place largely on the job but some instruction may be given through block and/or day release in an associated training school' (Bines, 1992). This approach, which has much in common with the apprenticeship model, sees training as the acquisition of 'cookbook' knowledge largely from practice manuals, combined with mastery of practice routines, and is provided mainly by experienced practitioners.

The introduction of the Project 2000 curriculum brought with it a move from the pre-technocratic to the technocratic model, which, as Bines pointed out, has become the pattern of education for most professions in recent years, and tends to take place in schools associated with, or incorporated into, institutions of higher education. She went on to suggest that:

> [the technocratic model] is characterised by the division of professional education into three main elements. The first comprises the development and transmission of a systematic knowledge base, largely, though not exclusively, based on contributing academic disciplines, such as the natural and social sciences, including both 'pure' and 'applied' dimensions. The second involves the interpretation and application of the knowledge base to practice... and may be based on theoretical models of practice, for example, 'the nursing process' in nurse education. The third element is the supervised practice in selected placements. (Bines, 1992)

These three elements correspond closely to the three components of professional knowledge suggested by Edgar Schein (1973) of basic science, applied science and technical skills, and describe a sequencing of the curriculum familiar to many Project 2000 teachers and students, from pure theory to applied theory to practice.

In my own school, which was among the first to implement the Project 2000 curriculum in 1989, this sequence was exemplified by the transition from a focus on health in the first part of the Common Foundation Programme to illness in the second part, at which time practice placements commenced. Thus, the students were first given the pure science of, say, the anatomy and physiology of the human body, often by academics from other departments. This was then *applied* to physical problems or illnesses by nurse tutors, and finally put into *practice* in the clinical setting. The fact that the students were presented with the theory before being placed in practice areas reinforced the dominance of theory over practice, that theory was something to be applied to practice. There was no notion of theory being generated *from* practice; it was a purely one-way process which reinforced the existing hierarchy.

Even in so-called 'progressive' schools which profess to have moved beyond the technocratic model, this sequencing from the pure sciences to their applied role in the causes and resolutions of ill health is still evident. In describing the nursing degree programme at Oxford Brookes University, a leader in progressive nurse education, Champion (1992) wrote of completely reshaping the syllabus 'putting health, people, families and community caring before illness or disturbance, hospitals and procedures', in other words, moving from biological, sociological and psychological theories of health and nursing to their practical application.

Similarly, Reed and Procter (1993) described a reflective course at the University of Northumbria in which the students are firstly given a grounding in 'basic skills and knowledge', including information retrieval skills, statistics, information technology, sociology, psychology and life science which is 'divorced from the world of practice'. Having acquired this knowledge and skill, the students are then encouraged to try it out in safe classroom settings, before finally applying and reflecting on it in real clinical situations. They continued:

> [these reflective strategies] assume that students will have gained, through reading, lectures, and experience an overall appreciation of the literature and thought relevant to the debate concerned, and *that their need is to learn how to use this knowledge*. (Reed and Proctor, 1993, my italics)

Thus, even in a course which professes to be based on the work of Schön, the purpose of reflective strategies is primarily for the students to learn to apply their body of formal theory and knowledge to practice settings rather than to extract theory from practice. I do not wish to criticise such syllabuses *per se*, only to point out that they contain within them the basic assumption of technical rationality that pure theory should (or must) be understood first, before being applied to nursing.

Technocratic education and the practicum

This technocratic model of nurse education makes great use of the practice setting or practicum, which is defined as 'a virtual world, relatively free of the pressures, distractions, and risks of the real one, to which, nevertheless, it refers' (Schön, 1987), and which in other departments of technical education such as engineering or biology, is usually the laboratory.

The laboratory has two functions in technocratic education: the first is to provide an environment where students can practice and develop skills in relative safety; and the second is to allow them to conduct experiments, the aim of which is not to generate new knowledge, but to confirm established theories. This second aim is of particular importance, since it reinforces the dominance of theory over practice by demonstrating the effectiveness of theory when applied to simulated real-life situations. For example, the engineering student will first learn the pure theory of metallurgy, will then learn to apply the theory to bridge design, and will finally utilise the laboratory to test and confirm that theory by building a bridge, or perhaps a model of a bridge. Furthermore, if the theory does not translate into practice, then there is assumed to be something wrong with the student rather than something wrong with the theory. If the bridge collapses, the theory is not called into question; rather, it is assumed either that the student had not gained a sufficient grasp of the theory, or that he did not have sufficient mastery of the skills of bridge building to apply it properly.

Similarly with nursing, the curriculum is organised so that practice follows theory, so that the student learns the theory in the classroom setting and then enters the practicum in order firstly to develop and practice the skills associated with that theory, and secondly to test and confirm that theory in practice. For example, the student learns the theory of counselling in a classroom setting, and may initially rehearse the associated skills with colleagues in the safety of the classroom. But eventually, he will try them out with real patients in real clinical settings, albeit under supervision in relatively controlled conditions. As in the previous engineering example, if his counselling intervention is effective, then the theory is confirmed. If it is ineffective, then according to the technocratic model of education, it is not because there is something wrong with the theory, but because there is something wrong with the way in which it was put into practice. If the student has difficulty in applying theory to practice as part of a practical assessment or examination, it is considered that it is the student and not the theory that has failed.

In nursing, however, a true practicum is very difficult to construct, and the working clinical environment is usually employed. The main disadvantage of a clinical environment from the point of view of technical education is that it cannot be fully controlled, and it is not, in Schön's words, 'free of pressures, distractions and risks'. In fact it is a combination of a practicum and an apprenticeship setting, and the aim of the clinically based teacher is therefore to make the clinical environment as much like a practicum or laboratory as she is able. She must ensure that the setting is controlled and as near 'perfect' as possible, and that practice is carried out 'by the book'. Her role is to demonstrate good practice by example, and to ensure that the 'messy' practice of real practitioners in real clinical areas does not contaminate the ideal laboratory setting. It could be argued, of course, that the clinical teacher is virtually extinct, but the current debate over the role of the link tutor and the lecturer practitioner would suggest that there is still a demand for the model clinical area in which students can observe and learn the ideals of nursing practice rather than the messy realities.

Post-technocratic education and the nurse–practitioner

To summarise, the aim of the prevalent technocratic model of nurse education is to produce 'knowledgeable doers', nurse–technicians who work from a sound empirical knowledge base. Nursing practice is grounded in formal theory generated through scientific research, and the student acquires a solid theoretical knowledge base before he is allowed into the practice area to apply it.

Schön (1987), however, has observed that this technocratic model of education is failing the professions, that 'what aspiring practitioners most need to learn, professional schools seem least able to teach', and Bines (1992) has highlighted several weaknesses in the technocratic model of education when applied to nursing and other professions. Firstly, she argued that 'there may be considerable variations in concepts of professional competence, the knowledge base transmitted, approaches to teaching both theory and practice, and the degrees of student choice', emphasising that, despite its claims, technocratic education does not result in a uniform curriculum. Secondly, she suggested that such a model can fragment learning into discrete and unrelated parts, including the separation of theory and practice. Finally, she claimed that the 'two-step application of knowledge to practice' implicit in this model does not reflect the true nature of professional knowledge and action, which is made up of messy and indeterminate situations.

This last point is precisely that being made in earlier chapters of this book. Technocratic education can never satisfy the needs of the nurse-practitioner, since she works within a very different framework of knowledge and theory from the nurse-technician. In particular, she is concerned with the generation of her own personal knowledge and informal theory, for which technocratic education makes no provision. What is required for the nurse-practitioner, then, is a model of education which ascribes as much importance to informal theory, theory generated out of practice, as it does to pure, formal theory.

Bines (1992) referred to models of this kind as post-technocratic. Such an approach to education 'is not yet a coherent or fully developed model, but it does include particular features, in particular the emphasis on the acquisition of professional competencies'. She pointed out that there is a great deal of disagreement over the term 'competencies', but that the usual definition is a behavioural one of being able to perform the activities within an occupation. In the example given earlier, this would entail being able to demonstrate a range of counselling interventions, and to explain and account for them from existing theory.

However, a truly post-technocratic model of education would view competencies not just as being able to perform within the parameters of existing theory, but to analyse, evaluate and reflect on one's own performance, and to generate new, informal micro theory out of that performance. This would entail abandoning the hierarchical relationship of theory to practice in which theory is learnt first and then applied to practice, in favour of the model referred to in Chapter 1 as nursing praxis, in which practice is not only informed by formal, scientific theory, but more importantly, by informal, personal theory which is generated out of practice itself.

The adoption of a post-technocratic model has a number of profound implications for nurse education. Firstly, the primary aim of education is not now seen as the transmission of knowledge and theory from teacher to student, but as the generation of knowledge and theory by the student himself. The role of the teacher is therefore very different from her role in the technocratic model, and the relationship between teacher and student is one of equals, or as equal as possible given the inevitable power relationship inherent in professional education.

Secondly, the curriculum does not progress from pure to applied science, but combines the two. Formal theory is still taught, but its position in the hierarchy of knowledge is secondary to that of informal theory generated out of practice. Furthermore, subject boundaries are broken down and formal theory is taught as an integrated body *as it applies to nursing*. And since it is recognised that formal theory is dynamic and ever changing, as much emphasis is placed on learning how to access knowledge and theory as on learning existing knowledge and theories (Dewey, 1916).

And thirdly, the practicum assumes a far greater importance and is seen in a different light. It is no longer a place where students go to try out the theories they have learned in the classroom, but rather it is the central focus of their education and a place where they generate new, personal knowledge and test out informal theory. Schön wrote of a new kind of reflective practicum in which:

> We will see students as having to learn a kind of reflection-in-action that goes beyond statable rules—not only by devising new methods of reasoning... but also by constructing and testing new categories of understanding, strategies of action, and ways of framing problems. (Schön, 1987)

This reflective practicum in turn requires a new kind of clinical teacher, whose job is not to impose order, structure and 'perfection' on the clinical area, to ensure that everything is done by the book, but rather to attempt, with the student, to make sense of the messy business of professional practice, to explore the limits of pure theory when applied to real-life practice situations, and to facilitate the student in reflection-on-action through supervision and critical incident analysis. The emphasis is therefore on her expertise as a teacher and facilitator of learning rather than as a clinician.

These issues must all be taken into account when designing a post-technocratic course to meet the needs of the nurse-practitioner. In addition, however, the course must satisfy two criteria: it must include a philosophy and methods of teaching and learning which enable the nurse to generate her own personal knowledge and informal theory; and it must locate that philosophy and those methods within a sound, practical and appropriate curriculum framework.

Philosophy and methods of teaching and learning for a post-technocratic model of nurse education

The nature of knowledge and learning

In order to arrive at a suitable philosophy of teaching and learning, we must begin by examining the very nature of knowledge itself. Traditional technocratic education views knowledge as existing 'out there' in the world, 'apart from, or outside of, the person who knows' (Chinn and Kramer, 1991), waiting to be uncovered by researchers and disseminated by educators. This school of thought argues, for example, that in physics the law of gravity existed before Newton discovered it, and in geometry Pythagoras' theorem has always existed, it is just that we did not know about it before Pythagoras.

Post-technocratic education, on the other hand, sees knowledge and theories as constructed or created rather than discovered, there being 'a fundamental unity between the knower and what is known' (Chinn and Kramer, 1991). The force we call gravity obviously predated Newton, but the *theory* of gravity and *knowledge* about gravity only exists in people's minds and on paper, and did not exist before 1687 when Newton invented it and wrote it down. Knowledge and theories are therefore created, in the case of nursing often by the nurse–practitioner herself, either by pure reason or by interacting with the physical world. As McNiff (1993) pointed out, 'in this sense knowing is an on-going act of creation by the person who makes a personal commitment to his own ability to know'.

That is not to say, of course, that all knowledge must be personally created by the knower. We saw in the previous chapter that a great deal of public knowledge already exists in Popper's 'World 3' in books and other physical media, more knowledge than any one person could possibly encounter in a lifetime, but it is in such a state of flux that it would be naive and short-sighted to attempt to teach very much of it to students. What is of far more value than learning facts and theories is for the student to learn how to learn, to learn how to gain access to World 3 knowledge for himself. Thus, both personal and public knowledge, both formal and informal theory, must be actively pursued. Formal, public theories and knowledge must be extracted by the student from the masses of irrelevant data in 'World 3', and informal, private theories and knowledge must be developed out of his own practice through reflection.

If learning is an active, creative process rather than the passive reception of knowledge handed down from above, then teaching will have a very different focus in post-technocratic education: thus, informal theory *cannot* be taught, and formal theory *should not* be taught. This view of teaching is reflected in Carl Rogers' assertion that: 'anything that can be taught to another is relatively inconsequential and has little or no significance on behaviour' (Rogers, 1957), a view supported by Boud *et al.*, who argued that:

> Only learners themselves can learn and only they can reflect on their own experiences. Teachers can intervene in various ways to assist, but they only have access to individuals' thoughts and feelings through what individuals choose to reveal about themselves. At this basic level the learner is in total control. (Boud *et al.*, 1985)

In addition to this new role for the teacher, any approach to post-technocratic education must also meet the requirements outlined earlier. It will be recalled that a post-technocratic model of nurse education has been described in this book as one in which:

- the role of the student is that of an equal partner in the generation of knowledge and theory;
- traditional boundaries between subjects are broken down, with learning structured according to its meaningfulness to the student;

- the practicum assumes a major importance, and is a place where knowledge is generated through a facilitated process of reflection-on-action, rather than being a place where it is tested.

A philosophy and method of education which appears to meet all of these criteria was developed by Carl Rogers during the 1950s, and is referred to as student-centred learning. It will now be briefly examined to determine whether it is suitable for the purpose of post-technocratic nurse education, either as Rogers described it or in a modified form.

Student-centred learning

The philosophy of student-centredness was developed by Rogers (1969, 1983) as an extension of his model of client-centred counselling, and shares many of its features. Both see the role of the facilitator, whether of counselling or learning, as being that of a non-directive enabler, and both consider the attitudes of the facilitator as the most important variables for a successful outcome. Rogers identified a threefold role for the facilitator of student-centred learning: to encourage learning firstly by optimising the physical resources of the classroom; secondly by structuring the learning activities of the group; and thirdly by setting the most conducive psychological climate for the learning to take place. Each of these will now be briefly examined in turn.

Optimising the physical resources of the classroom

With regard to this first role, Rogers referred not only to the usual academic resources such as books, articles, work space, laboratories, tools, maps, films, and so on, but also to human resources, most importantly the teacher herself. The teacher:

> Makes himself and his special knowledge and experience clearly available to the students, but he does not impose himself on them. He outlines the particular ways in which he feels he is most competent, and they can call on him for anything he is able to give. But this is an offer of himself as a resource and the degree to which he is used is up to the students. (Rogers, 1969)

The teacher is therefore a resource to be called upon by the students as and when required. She does not seek to direct them, but is there when needed, to be employed as a tool in much the same way as a reference book. This is clearly a far more passive and unobtrusive role than that traditionally associated with nurse education.

Structuring the learning activities of the group

Turning to the second role, Rogers suggested several ways in which learning activities might be structured, including the use of learning contracts, dividing the class into small functional, self-motivated groups, the use of simulation exercises, the use of encounter groups, and the use of self-evaluation, and these are all useful and relevant techniques in post-technocratic education. He argued against lectures and other direct teaching methods; indeed he saw no benefit in the practice of teaching at all, and described himself as a facilitator of learning rather than as a teacher. This is in sharp contrast to the traditional higher education model of teaching through lectures, and has more in common with pre-Project 2000 curricula.

Setting a psychological climate conducive to learning

Regarding this third role of the facilitator of learning, much of the success or failure of the learning experience depends on the qualities or attitudes that the facilitator displays as a person, and on the relationship that she has with her students. Rogers drew on his extensive work in counselling and psychotherapy to suggest that the attitudes which bring about learning when held by the teacher are the same as those which bring about therapeutic change when held by the counsellor, namely genuineness, respect and empathy.

The attitude of genuineness in the educational context involves the teacher in recognising her feelings as she is experiencing them, and communicating them to her students. In short, it means being herself and entering into an honest and meaningful relationship with her students. Rogers pointed out that this might mean being enthusiastic, being bored, being interested or being angry. Again, this is in sharp contrast to how many teachers behave with their students in hiding behind a mask or façade and putting on an act or performance.

The attitude of respect involves the teacher prizing her students, their feelings and their opinions. It means accepting her students as individuals in their own right and adopting a positive attitude towards them. It might seem on first sight that this attitude conflicts with the attitude of genuineness. For example, the teacher might feel angry with a student who repeatedly disrupts her classes. How is she to genuinely express her feelings of anger while at the same time maintaining a positive attitude towards the student? This seeming dilemma is resolved by the teacher expressing anger at her student's behaviour whilst continuing to respect the student as a person, regardless of his imperfections. It is an attitude of 'I like and value you but I don't like what you are doing', or as Rogers (1983) wrote: 'She can like or dislike a student product without implying that it is objectively good or bad or that the student is good or bad'.

The attitude of empathy is the ability to understand the student's reactions from the inside, the awareness of how the educational process appears to the student. Rogers claimed that the students' experience of feeling understood is a powerful factor in the process of learning, but that, as with the former two attitudes, it is so rare as to be almost absent from most classroom situations. Other qualities of the facilitator which Rogers identified as contributing to an effective psychological climate include a trust in the human organism and its tendencies towards growth, discovery, learning and self-actualisation, and the ability to live with uncertainty and take risks.

Rogers summed up the role of the facilitator of learning with a list of ten guidelines which are summarised below:

1. The facilitator has much to do with setting the initial mood or climate of the group or class experience;
2. The facilitator helps to elicit and clarify the purposes of the individuals in the class as well as the more general purposes of the group;
3. He relies upon the desire of each student to implement those purposes which have meaning for him, as the motivational force behind significant learning;

4. He endeavours to organize and make easily available the widest possible range of resources for learning;
5. He regards himself as a flexible resource to be utilized by the group;
6. In responding to expressions in the classroom group, he accepts both the intellectual content and the emotionalized attitudes, endeavouring to give each aspect the approximate degree of emphasis which it has for the individual or the group;
7. As the acceptant classroom climate becomes established, the facilitator is able increasingly to become a participant learner, a member of the group, expressing his views as those of one individual only;
8. He takes the initiative in sharing himself with the group — his feelings as well as his thoughts — in ways which do not demand nor impose but represent simply a personal sharing which students may take or leave;
9. Throughout the classroom experience, he remains alert to the expressions indicative of deep or strong feelings;
10. In his functioning as a facilitator of learning, the leader endeavours to recognize and accept his own limitations.

(from Rogers, 1969)

Student-centred courses clearly differ from traditional courses in higher education in a number of ways, and would appear to be particularly appropriate to the needs of the student nurse–practitioner who is an active, creative learner and generator of knowledge and theory. Student-centred courses are as much concerned with process as they are with content, with the 'how' of learning as well as with the 'what', and both process and content can be tailored to the individual needs of the student through negotiated learning contracts.

The role of the teacher is also very different. She is a facilitator, an organiser of resources and she is herself a resource. Her job is to set the psychological climate for effective learning and to suggest and facilitate alternative educational interventions such as simulation exercises, role-play, encounter groups and individual and group projects. But ultimately, it is the student who must take responsibility for his own learning, since:

thinking, decision making, problem solving, autonomous nurses will never result from courses where the thinking, decision making, problem solving and autonomy are mainly the responsibility of the course planners and teachers. Autonomous practitioners grow from autonomous students, and autonomous students are students who have a major part to play in what and how they are to learn. (Rolfe and Jasper, 1993)

Criticisms of student-centred learning

A number of criticisms have been levelled at student-centred courses over the years, both on political and on educational grounds. On the political front, some critics have argued that there is little place for an approach which originated in the 'financially secure' 1960s in these days of cutbacks and a move towards larger class sizes in higher education. However, it is a common misunderstanding of student-centred methods that they require high teacher–student ratios and increased resources to work properly. It must be emphasised that the lecture method is not the only way to teach large numbers of students, and many alternatives have been developed, including student-facilitated groups and individual and group project work.

What *is* required, though, is regular one-to-one contact between student and teacher to plan and negotiate learning objectives to support the student in achieving those objectives, and to check that they are being met. However, *any* well-resourced course, whether student-centred or traditional, should be able to offer regular tutorials of some kind, and the resourcing issues for a student-centred course are therefore no greater than for any other course.

It has also been argued that today's political climate militates against what are still seen by some as experimental teaching methods. Certainly, there has been a move during the 1990s to return to more traditional educational approaches in primary and secondary education, and it could be argued that in a market economy we should stick with tried and tested methods in nurse education as well. There is no easy answer to this objection, which appears to be based on rational grounds, but which is actually an ideological point. In fact, student-centred methods have been well researched over the past 40 years, and cannot really be described either as experimental or as untried and untested. Therefore, I can only restate my belief that student-centred courses produce thinking, decision-making autonomous nurses, and the real issue is whether or not the profession sees these as better value for money than the compliant, non-questioning variety.

The educational objections to student-centred courses are rather more substantial, and come not only from educational traditionalists, but also from more progressive writers. A number of these objections have been raised by Reed and Procter (1993), who advocate a reflective approach to nurse education, but reject the student-centred philosophy. Each of their objections will now be examined in turn.

Firstly, they invoke the objection that many students put forward on first being introduced to a student-centred curriculum: that 'students, almost by definition, cannot determine their own learning, because they do not know what they need to know, and therefore their learning must be guided' (Reed and Procter, 1993). On first sight, this objection appears persuasive, indeed, it seems almost paradoxical for students to be able to know what they need to know before they actually know it!

However, this seeming paradox is based on two different meanings of the verb 'to know', and would not present as a problem in many other languages which distinguish between knowing as obtaining knowledge, and knowing as being acquainted with a person or object. Thus the Germans have the verbs *wissen* and *kennen*, and the French have *savoir* and *connaître*. Bearing this in mind, there is no logical reason why students cannot be *acquainted* with what they need to know before they actually know it — indeed, that is one purpose of a syllabus. It is quite conceivable, therefore, for a student to be able to identify, for example, the need to know how to carry out mouthcare without actually knowing how to do it, and the student-centred approach argues that much of what students identify as important knowledge comes directly from their clinical experiences.

A second objection put forward by Reed and Procter is that 'many of the texts on student-centred learning emphasise the importance of allowing students to make their own decisions about how to solve problems' and that within this problem-solving framework 'students are expected to make mistakes, which will become a focus for further learning'. This, they argue, is simply not possible in clinical areas, since to make mistakes might put patients at risk, a difficulty which arises partly from the lack of access by most students to a laboratory-type practicum. Therefore, 'students can't learn from their mistakes, but must accept the decision of the qualified nurse even if they are not yet able to understand it' (Reed and Proctor, 1993), thus necessitating a didactic approach to learning.

However, this objection displays a misconception of the problem-solving method employed in many practical fields, including nursing, which is not based on a kind of trial and error and learning from mistakes, but on a reflexive cycle of theory generation and hypothesis testing, referred to in this book as hypothetico-abductivism. Indeed, the assessment, planning, implementation and evaluation phases of the nursing process follow a similar cycle. The essence of student-centred learning is not of learning from mistakes, but of the facilitator of learning working with each individual student to enable him to identify his own individual learning needs, to plan and implement ways of meeting those needs, and to evaluate the outcomes. Care-giving can always be improved, and evaluating and improving care is not the same as learning from mistakes.

Thirdly, Reed and Procter argue that a student-centred curriculum in which students identify their own learning needs is rather hit-and-miss, and is likely to miss out much of the hidden, tacit knowledge of expert practitioners. However, the exact opposite is true, and it is more likely that tacit, contextual knowledge and skills will be overlooked in a traditional tutor-directed course where the curriculum writers are not currently full-time practising nurses. Tacit knowledge, by definition, is very difficult to teach in a formal, didactic way, and by identifying problems from their own practice as they arise, students are far more likely to get in touch with the real issues of nursing and their real life, 'messy' solutions.

And fourthly, they argue that clinical placements are too unstructured and unpredictable to offer the kind of graded exposure to the realities of practice that is required of a student-centred course. However, it is a common mistake to think of student-centred learning as requiring the kind of graded exposure from simple to complex problems, or from one set of patient problems to another as is required with technical education. The whole point of student-centred learning is that the students will structure their own individual learning programmes, in consultation with their facilitator of learning and in response to their own individual clinical needs, rather than having an artificial structure imposed on them from above.

Reflection-on-action

Despite a number of objections, a student-centred curriculum is not only a practical and feasible approach to learning, but is possibly the most appropriate approach for student nurse-practitioners. However, Rogers was not directly concerned with the education of practice-based professionals, and so did not consider the special educational problems associated with the relationship between theory and practice. It is hardly surprising, therefore, that learning through reflection-on-action is not specifically addressed by Rogers as a student-centred learning technique. Nevertheless, for the nurse-practitioner it is probably the most important learning method of all, since it represents the most straightforward and direct means of generating knowledge and theory out of practice. Fortunately, the conditions necessary for reflection to take place are remarkably similar to those described by Rogers, since:

> One of the key features of self-reflection is the need for people to have the freedom to make a genuine choice for themselves rather than conform to the influence of the teacher or other students. For this to happen... there must be a structure which allows equal power relationships between group members, including the teacher or facilitator, if the freedom to choose is to be a valid one. (Boud *et al.*, 1985)

It should be possible, then, to integrate the learning technique of reflection-on-action into a student-centred philosophy of learning.

Reflection-on-action has become very popular in nursing in the 1990s, but there is still a great deal of confusion over its aims and purpose. A typical definition of reflection is:

> The process of internally examining and exploring an issue of concern, triggered by an experience, which creates and clarifies meaning in terms of self, and which results in a changed conceptual perspective. (Boyd and Fales, 1983)

This definition makes the important point that the goal of reflection is not simply to improve practice, but to change the way in which practice is conceptualised. Reflective practice should not short-circuit the intellect. It is not enough to merely change our nursing interventions with a particular patient as a result of reflecting on them. Changes in practice must be mediated by changes to our personal knowledge base and our network of informal theory, and should take in the whole of the nursing praxis cycle, including the stages of knowledge generation and theory construction. It is only in this way that our experiences are turned into knowledge and stored as paradigm cases rather than being utilised once, in one specific situation, before being lost forever.

However, although the above definition is useful, by focusing on issues of concern it suggests that reflection is a technique to be employed only in unusual or critical situations rather than as an everyday method of knowledge and theory generation. A better definition comes from Fitzgerald, who claimed:

> Reflection on action is the retrospective contemplation of practice undertaken in order to uncover the knowledge used in a particular situation, by analysing and interpreting the information recalled. (Fitzgerald, 1994)

For our requirements, then, reflection-on-action is an everyday part of nursing life, with the aim of turning experience into knowledge through a formal process which might involve working alone on journal entries, working with peers on critical incident analysis, or working with a clinical supervisor. Whatever methods are employed, the purpose of reflection-on-action is to generate what Benner referred to as a repertoire of paradigm cases which can be drawn upon in future clinical situations. This knowledge is not generalisable, and is personal to the practitioner who generated it. Nevertheless, it is an important source of knowledge and theory for the nurse–practitioner, possibly more so than the formal, shared knowledge from the public domain.

So how does reflection-on-action as an educational process differ from reflection-on-action as a research method which was discussed in the previous chapter? The short answer is that there is no difference; research and education are both concerned with the generation of knowledge and theories, and therefore, for the nurse–practitioner, education and research are one and the same. Whether the student is doing research or whether he is doing education, he is engaged in the same process, the process of creating knowledge and building theory. This is equally true for public knowledge and formal theory as it is for personal knowledge and informal theory, since as we have seen, the nurse–practitioner is more interested in the process of learning than in the *content*. In other words, she is concerned with learning how to learn, with how to gain access to information rather than with attempting to memorise it, and this is as much a research technique as reflection-on-action or empirical scientific methods.

To summarise, a philosophy for teaching the nurse–practitioner borrowing heavily from the work of Rogers has been outlined. This student-centred approach is particularly concerned with the facilitative attitudes of the teacher and with the degree of control exerted by the students over their own learning, both in terms of process and content. It rejects formal teaching methods as inappropriate, relying instead on small group work, directed individual study and learning contracts. It also draws extensively on the method of reflection-on-action, and sees the students as generators of their own knowledge and theories.

Curriculum framework for a post-technocratic model of nurse education

The reflective spiral curriculum

In order to construct a coherent and workable model of post-technocratic nurse education, the above philosophy and teaching methods need to be located within a sound, practical and appropriate curriculum framework. We have seen that traditional Project 2000 curricula tend to follow the technocratic

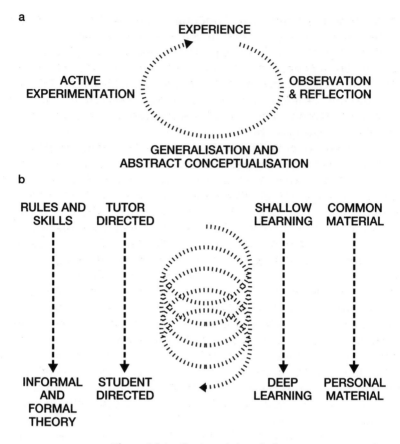

Figure 3.1 A reflective spiral curriculum

model of education, progressing from pure theory to applied theory to practice in a linear, hierarchical fashion. However, this type of curriculum model is of little use in the education of the nurse-practitioner, since for her, theory and practice do not conform to a linear relationship, but to a cyclical one, where theory is constructed from practice and is then applied back into practice in a reflective learning cycle (Kolb and Fry, 1975) (Figure 3.1a).

It might appear possible, then, to adopt this reflective cycle as an alternative curriculum model to the linear models on which most Project 2000 courses are based. However, the problem with cyclical models is that, by definition, they lack any real notion of progression. If a cyclical model is to be of any use, therefore, it must account for the fact that each revolution around the cycle takes place at ever deeper levels, and this can be achieved by expanding the two-dimensional cycle into the third dimension, in other words, by transforming the cycle into a spiral (Figure 3.1b).

The model of the spiral curriculum, first proposed by Brunner (1966), is ideally suited to a course such as the one being described here, where students are introduced into practice areas very early on. Unlike traditional 'block and placement' models where the students are provided with the theory relating to a particular aspect of nursing, which they then attempt to apply in a relevant placement, a spiral curriculum covers a broad expanse of curricular content very quickly and on a fairly superficial level. The content is then periodically revisited at ever deeper and more detailed levels as the course progresses. The students are therefore equipped very early in the course with a broad span of albeit fairly shallow knowledge which they can apply to a variety of nursing situations rather than just to one specific clinical area.

In contrast to Brunner's traditional spiral model, the *reflective* spiral curriculum shown in Figure 3.1 is structured around informal rather than formal theory, and personal rather than public knowledge, and begins with very little, if any, theory at all. The first time around the spiral is practice-focused, and students will be taught the procedural rules and simple skills which they will need in order to survive, and possibly function at a very basic level, in *any* clinical setting. This is truly common foundational material, consisting of what Benner (1984) described as 'context-free rules to guide action', basic nursing and communication skills, and skills of reflection. The students then apply those rules and practice those basic skills in clinical settings and reflect on their experiences, thereby generating very basic personal knowledge.

Each time the student travels round the cycle from experience to reflection to conceptualisation to experimentation and back to experience, his experiences become more clinical and more meaningful, his reflections are more profound, the knowledge that is generated is deeper, he has more control over process and content, and requires less direct supervision. Furthermore, in the early stages of the course, the material generated through reflection, although personal to the students, is likely to be common to most of them, since the students are engaging in practice at a fairly superficial level and many of the issues raised are likely to be issues that concern all of them. As the course progresses and the students are allowed more direction over the process and content of their learning, the knowledge and theory generated from reflection-on-action will become far more individual and personal to particular students. Furthermore, their practice progresses from being the non-contextualised rule-governed behaviour of the novice to the 'aspect' based practice of the advanced beginner, where:

> aspects, in contrast to the measurable, context-free attributes or the procedural lists of things to do that are learned and used by the beginner, require prior experience in actual situations for recognition. (Benner, 1984)

Formal theory and research-based knowledge is introduced some way into the course to support and reinforce personal knowledge and to assist in the generation of informal theory. Furthermore, in a student-centred reflective spiral curriculum, the formal theory relevant to each individual student will be identified and negotiated through learning contracts, and it will be the responsibility of the student to acquire it by the most appropriate means.

Thus, in a traditional 'block and placement' nursing curriculum, formal theory is taught first and is then applied to practice, and if reflective techniques *are* used, the personal knowledge and paradigm cases generated by reflection-on-action are employed to support and confirm the formal theory. In contrast, in the reflective spiral curriculum, procedural rules and basic skills are taught first, followed by the generation of personal knowledge through reflection, with formal theory being employed to support the students' own informal theory. The traditional technical educational sequence of a progression from theory to practice is therefore reversed in the reflective spiral curriculum, and the hierarchy of basic science, applied science and technical skills is turned on its head.

Reflective spirals can be of any size. It is possible on the one hand to construct a reflective spiral around a single incident, which can be revisited at ever deeper and more personal levels. For example, a student's experience of the death of a patient he was caring for can be initially addressed by considering the procedures and basic skills necessary to deal with the situation, before employing the technique of reflection-on-action to examine firstly the issues common to all deaths and bereavements, then exploring the deeper and more personal issues. Finally, the search for formal theory relating to death and bereavement can be facilitated and employed in the construction of informal theory relating to this particular patient.

At the other extreme, a reflective spiral can encompass a whole syllabus, but in our experience, the most practical size for the spiral is the 'theme' (Jasper and Rolfe, 1993; Rolfe and Jasper, 1993). A theme is a self-contained unit within the syllabus which seeks to meet specific learning outcomes, and ideally represents between 1 week and 1 month of course material. Themes offer an ideal opportunity to cut across traditional subject disciplines and integrate a number of different perspectives on a single issue.

An example of a theme might be 'communication', where students would initially learn basic communication skills and procedural rules which they would then be expected to apply in clinical settings and reflect on through journals, clinical supervision and critical incident analysis. Preliminary reflections are likely to be fairly superficial, and would probably address issues of common concern to the whole group, for example, 'what do I say on first meeting a patient?'. By applying the personal knowledge generated from these reflections back into practice, deeper and more personal communications issues would be encountered, and the students would steer their learning along individual pathways of direct relevance to their current clinical placements and personal needs.

Finally, students would be facilitated to seek out formal theory relating to the issues identified in their reflection-on-action, and would be encouraged to synthesise relevant material from a variety of sociological, psychological, biological and philosophical sources into a body of personalised knowledge, theory and skills. Towards the end of the course, once the students had started to build up a repertoire of paradigm cases and had gained some experience in the construction of informal theory, they would be encouraged to generate and test out hypotheses in the clinical situation, thereby completing the cycle of nursing praxis. An example of a reflective spiral curriculum based on themes is presented in Part 2 of this book.

The problem of prescribed syllabus material

A particular problem with the reflective spiral curriculum model in professional education is in reconciling the student-directed content of the course with the requirements demanded by higher education and the constraints imposed by a syllabus for professional training. Clearly there is a body of common skills, public knowledge and formal theory which all nurses must possess if they are to be safe, competent practitioners, and any pre-registration course for nurses must ensure that this material is included.

The reflective spiral makes provision for the introduction of public knowledge and formal theory at the deeper levels, but the imposition from outside and above of course material runs counter to the philosophy of student-centred learning and reflec-tion-on-action, and raises issues of professional paternalism and clinical relevance. If curriculum is 'a selection from culture' (Lawton, 1980), then perhaps there is a need to examine the motives of those educationalists who are doing the selecting. In particular, is the selection of material being made in the best interests of the patients being cared for by the students, or in the interests of a profession committed to an outdated and inappro-priate technical rationality model of nursing? If the latter, then the students might have difficulty in seeing the relevance and application of externally imposed syllabus material to clinical work, and as educationalists have demonstrated (Maddox, 1963; Rogers, 1969, 1983), this is not conducive to learning, and will only serve to widen the theory–practice gap.

For example, the syllabus might require students to study theoretical models of nursing. If the student does not identify the need for a model in his own practice, and if the clinical areas he is working in do not employ models to structure care, then it is unlikely that the issue of nursing models will ever arise for that student. If this situation is only experienced by a few students, then ways must be found to ensure that the relevant material is covered. If, however, it is a situation common to all the students, then questions should be raised as to the reasons for introducing material into the syllabus that is not seen as relevant either by students or by practising nurses. However, in the short term, prescribed syllabus material must be covered, whether relevant or not.

The problem for the nurse tutor wishing to facilitate a student-centred course within a reflective spiral curriculum is therefore one of allowing the students to identify their own learning needs while at the same time ensuring that the prescribed syllabus material is covered. It could be argued that if the prescribed syllabus material is truly relevant to nursing, then it will be precisely this material that the students will identify through reflection-on-action. This requires a certain faith in the students, and a much greater faith in the syllabus writers. However, there will inevitably be material included in the syllabus which some students do not identify as relevant and ongoing issues, and the problem is therefore how this material can be introduced in a student-centred manner which is sensitive to the needs of each individual.

One approach to individualising common core material has been suggested by Jane Abercrombie, who proposed the use of free group discussions, in which small groups of eight to ten students are presented with written, audio or visual material which they study alone for a set period before discussing it as a group. Free group discussions offer a practical and viable alternative to the lecture, allowing for greater flexibility in the presentation of core material, since:

> In giving a lecture, the teacher organises the material in such a way that it will, he hopes, be comprehended or assimilated in roughly the way he intends it should be. Ideally, then, if he is successful, all the students receive the same information, and it is the information he intended they should receive. In free group discussion, on the other hand, the students are presented with the same information (for example, two radiographs or an account of an experiment), but it soon becomes clear that they do not extract the same information from it, and learning depends on the fact that each extracts something different. (Abercrombie, 1979)

This method allows each individual student to extract personal information of relevance to his own practice-based experience and his own particular interests from common, prescribed syllabus material, thereby reconciling the demands of a professional syllabus with the needs of the individual student. For example, the group might be given a theoretical paper on sleep and sleeping problems, which each individual student will interpret and utilise in relation to his own current clinical needs and experiences. These different perspectives would then be shared and debated by the group, and each individual could build up a global picture of sleeping problems from a wide variety of clinical perspectives.

A second method of ensuring individual relevance is to employ learning contracts within a framework of clinical or theoretical objectives, so that all the students are required to meet the same learning outcomes, but can negotiate with the tutor the exact content and process which will suit their specific learning needs. For example, all students undertaking a Common Foundation Programme might be required to meet theoretical and practical objectives relating to sleep; however, these objectives will have a different focus depending on the client group that the student is currently working with. For example, a student on a surgical ward might be faced with the problem of patients who find it difficult to sleep the night before surgery. He could explore the relationship between sleep and insomnia, and investigate ways of helping the patients deal with their anxiety and thus promote sleep without medication. On the other hand, a student working on an acute psychiatric ward might be nursing a patient suffering from depression, and would thus be faced with an entirely different set of sleep-related problems to resolve. In this way, the prescribed content of the syllabus is covered, but at different times by different students, and in a way that meshes with the current focus of their reflection-on-action.

Student-centred assessment and the reflective spiral curriculum

Gibbs (1992) considered assessment to be the key element in a successful student-centred course, and the most important factor in setting the learning culture. There is a considerable amount of evidence that assessment systems dominate what students are oriented towards in their learning. Even where lecturers say that they want students to be creative and thoughtful, students often recognise that what is really necessary, or at least what is sufficient, is to memorise (Gibbs, 1992). In a truly student-centred reflective spiral curriculum, there would be no examinations and all assessment would be formative and tailored to the learning needs of individual students, with self and peer assessment featuring strongly. However, the full implementation of self and peer assessment presents problems for a course whose aim is to control and restrict entry to a profession, and where a regulating body sets out precise assessment guidelines. It is important, therefore, to distinguish between formative and summative applications of self and peer assessment. Whereas the former is employed with great success in many courses for professionals in the form of reflective diaries, critical incident work, role-play, and a host of other techniques, self and peer *summative* assessment is fraught with difficulty. Thus, although some Project 2000 courses are beginning to introduce elements of summative self and peer assessment, its success relies heavily on acceptance and co-operation by the students, and this in turn depends on the students seeing self and peer assessment as being meaningfully integrated into the assessment structure, and as having a real bearing on their overall grade.

However, if the nursing profession wishes to continue to regulate its membership, self and peer assessment can never play more than a small part in the total summative schedule. I therefore feel it to be dishonest to allow students to believe that they have a real and meaningful say in whether they qualify as nurses, when in fact their contribution to the process is necessarily marginal.

An alternative and more realistic approach would be to concentrate on making the assessment process as clinically relevant to the students as possible, and to give them real choices in the material they are assessed on. This approach is far more in keeping with a reflective spiral curriculum where students will be learning different material, in different sequences, and at different speeds. Gibbs (1992) made a number of useful suggestions in this area, including greater involvement of students in the design of assessments and the choice of assessment tasks through the use of contracts; integrating assessment into the learning process; and setting assessed tasks which are similar to 'real world' situations and problems. The use of portfolios and structured workbooks is a particularly powerful tool in responding to all the above suggestions, and is outlined fully in Part 2 of the book.

This approach to assessment is particularly problematic, however, when it comes to formal examinations, which the ENB still insists on as part of pre-registration training. They outline four conditions which must be met (ENB, 1990), namely:

• All students must undertake the same examination(s).
• The examination(s) must be taken under controlled conditions.
• The examination(s) must be completed within a predetermined time period which should be sufficient to enable candidates to complete the examination.
• The specific content of the activity to be undertaken must not be known by students prior to the commencement of the examination(s).

Beyond these conditions, little guidance is given regarding structure, although the ENB appears to be encouraging alternatives to the old state final exam format by suggesting that students may be given general topic material in advance, and by allowing students access to information during the exam. With regard to content, the exam must test 'the depth of theoretical knowledge and concepts applied to practice' (ENB, 1990).

The challenge for the assessor is to produce individualised, clinically relevant examinations which test for depth of knowledge in a student-centred way, and yet fall within the ENB guidelines. As a framework for writing an examination which satisfies both the philosophy of the reflective spiral curriculum and the requirements of the ENB, I have constructed a set of criteria which includes the following:

• The exam should test the depth of theoretical knowledge and concepts, that is, it should be a test of problem solving

and higher order cognitive abilities and should not be merely a measure of recall or memory.
- It should test knowledge as applied to practice, that is, it should have meaning and relevance to clinical work rather than being a dry academic exercise.
- It should be flexible enough to assess each student on the unique and personal learning objectives that he has negotiated with his tutor.
- It should be responsive to the curriculum rather than determining syllabus material. In other words, the content of the exam should reflect what the students have learnt rather than the course being designed to get the students through the exam.

My colleagues and I have devised a number of approaches to examinations based on these criteria. The one to be outlined here is the end of CFP exam for a reflective spiral course based on the principles described earlier in the chapter, and presented more fully in Part 2 of this book. In this course, the students have a great deal of flexibility in pursuing issues of relevance to their specific work with the patients they are nursing. Thus, not only are they generating a great deal of personal knowledge and theory through reflection-on-action, but much of their formal, public theory and knowledge is individual to each of them. Furthermore, the depth and breadth to which that material is explored is very much at the discretion of the students, and depends on their patients' individual needs. The challenge, therefore, was to construct an examination which met the ENB specification of being the same for each candidate, whilst acknowledging that each candidate had developed and pursued their own unique programme of learning.

The solution was to write a paper containing very general questions which the student had to answer in relation to one of his own patients on whom he had been writing a portfolio. For example, the student might be required to discuss the problems of hospital related stress *as it applies to his patient*. It is clear that different students will raise different issues depending on the situation and diagnosis of the patient, and that these issues will be addressed at different levels. There is ample opportunity for the student to introduce his own informal theory from his reflection-on-action, to construct theory out of practice, and to apply it back into practice.

It can be seen that this very simple approach elegantly meets the above four criteria, since it clearly assesses depth of knowledge applied to clinical situations, it is geared to assessing the individual learning objectives negotiated by each student at the appropriate level, and the students are free to direct their learning according to their own needs and the needs of their patients, rather than towards covering the narrow and prescribed range of material necessary to pass a traditional examination.

The reflective spiral curriculum and nursing praxis

It might be useful at this stage to review the process of the reflective spiral curriculum for pre-registration nurse education in relation to nursing praxis and the requirements of the nurse–practitioner. It will be recalled that the first stage of the process is to provide the new student with a basic repertoire of procedural rules and skills for practice, and to introduce him into the clinical area very early in his training. The starting point of the reflective spiral curriculum is thus with practice, albeit at a very basic and rudimentary level (Figure 3.2a).

The second stage is to facilitate the student to reflect on his clinical experiences by employing the techniques of reflection-on-action and critical incident analysis, and in this way to begin to construct a body of personal knowledge and experience which will later grow into a situational repertoire of paradigm cases and tacit knowledge (Figure 3.2b).

In the third stage, this body of personal knowledge and experience begins to be turned into informal theory that can be employed to generate and test hypotheses (Figure 3.2c). This is the most difficult part of the process and requires high level cognitive skills of analysis and synthesis. It involves the student in examining a nurse–patient interaction or a patient's response to a nursing intervention, asking *why* the patient responded in a particular way. It will involve the application not only of personal knowledge and past paradigm cases, but also of formal theory and empirical research.

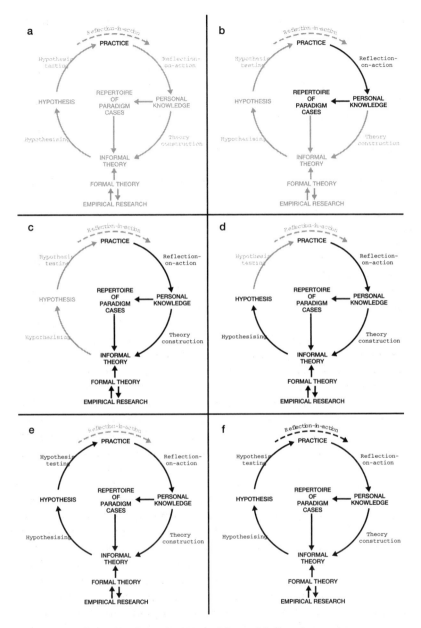

Figure 3.2 Nurse education and the model of nursing praxis

Take as an example a student who has read research reports suggesting that giving information to patients about forthcoming surgery can, in some cases, lead to improved post-operative recovery. He decides to implement the findings with his own patient, only to find that the patient becomes distressed and asks to terminate the discussion. The student is then faced with the task of making sense of this personal experience and turning it into a theory that will explain the behaviour of this particular patient in this situation.

It might be, for example, that the patient responded as he did because of the way in which the student presented the information, his reaction might have been a function of his personality, or it might have been as a result of a previous experience in hospital. By reflecting on his encounter with the patient during clinical supervision, the student decides that the latter theory is the most probable in this case.

The fourth stage is for the student to apply this informal theory to practice by generating hypotheses and questions from his reflection-on-action (Figure 3.2d) to be tested out in real practice situations (Figure 3.2e). The student decides to test out the theory that the patient's response was as a result of past experiences, and attempts on his next visit to the ward to talk to the patient about previous visits to hospital. If it appears that this hypothesis is incorrect, then his further reflection-on-action might lead him to generate a hypothesis based on the theory that the information was delivered in an untherapeutic way, and then to test that out in practice, and so on, until he finds a theory which 'fits' the situation. It should be noted that this is not blind 'trial and error', but a systematic process of hypothesis construction and testing based on the logical process of hypothetico-abductivism.

It can be seen from Figure 3.2f that the reflective spiral curriculum process leaves the model of nursing praxis incomplete. The student has learnt to apply informal theory generated from his reflection-on-action to his practice, but he is unable to complete the cycle of reflection-*in*-action by modifying his informal theory *on the spot* as a result of that practice. Theory building therefore only takes place in the classroom after the event. The student enters a practice situation armed with a body of formal and informal theory, but has no way of adding to that theory during his clinical encounter with the patient. He can test previously generated hypotheses in practice, but cannot then modify his informal theory as a result, nor can he construct new hypotheses until he reflects on his practice later in the classroom. He is therefore unable to carry out on-the-spot experimenting.

Post-registration education for the nurse–practitioner

Education for expertise

By the end of his pre-registration nurse training, the student on a reflective spiral course should have reached Benner's second stage of Advanced Beginner. Nurses at this stage are:

> ones who can demonstrate marginally acceptable performance, ones who have coped with enough real situations to note (or to have pointed out to them by a mentor) the recurring meaningful situational components that are termed 'aspects of the situation'. (Benner, 1984)

More importantly, however, the reflective spiral course equips the student to proceed through Benner's stages to the fifth and final stage of expert. The expert, for Benner, is a nurse who:

> with an enormous background of experience, now has an intuitive grasp of each situation and zeroes in on the accurate region of the problem without wasteful consideration of a large range of unfruitful, alternative diagnoses and solutions. (Benner, 1984)

Accelerated progress to the stage of expert, which would normally take many years, is possible because, as Benner pointed out, 'experience, as the word is used here, does not refer to the mere passage of time or longevity', and 'there is a leap, a discontinuity, between the competent level and the proficient and expert levels'. Making this leap involves learning to employ tacit knowledge, what Benner referred to as intuitive grasp, rather than explicit procedural rules. But whereas it would normally take a great deal of time, experience and confidence to begin to trust and rely on tacit, personal knowledge and theory, the reflective spiral curriculum introduces techniques for generating it early on, and stresses its importance throughout the course. Graduates from reflective spiral courses therefore employ reflection-on-action and informal theory building as a normal part of their everyday practice, and are relying on their personal, tacit knowledge or intuitive grasp almost from day one. The only outstanding condition for expertise, therefore, is the building up of a repertoire of paradigm cases.

Beyond the expert practitioner

It has been argued that the graduate from a reflective spiral course is equipped to reach the level of expert in a relatively short space of time. However, such a course in itself does not allow the student to fully meet the criteria described in Chapter 1 for a nurse–practitioner, since his training has not provided him with the final link in the cycle of nursing praxis (Figure 3.2f), namely, the ability to carry out reflection-in-action. Whereas the pre-registration course outlined above could be described as *reflective* education, post-basic courses would need to focus on *reflexive* education that would enable the nurse to build and modify theory *during* the therapeutic encounter through on-the-spot experimenting rather than afterwards through reflection-on-action. The whole aim of post-basic nurse–practitioner education, then, is to make the final link from practice back to informal theory, thereby completing the cycle of reflection-in-action, and this takes the nurse–practitioner beyond Benner's fifth level of expert.

Expertise, for Benner, is concerned with working intuitively, with responding to practice situations from a body of personal, tacit knowledge, a repertoire of past paradigm cases. Dreyfus and Dreyfus described this expertise in terms of the experienced performer, who:

> is no longer aware of features and rules, and his/her performance becomes fluid and flexible and highly proficient. The chess player develops a feel for the game; the language learner becomes fluent; the pilot stops feeling that he/she is flying the plane and simply feels that he/she is flying. (Dreyfus and Dreyfus, 1977)

This notion of 'getting the feel' for an activity, of being able to do it almost without thinking will be familiar to all experienced car drivers or typists, and is referred to by psychologists as 'chunking'. Chunking is the process by which larger and larger units of behaviour or cognition come to be seen holistically as a single thought or action.

> To the novice, typing proceeds letter by letter; to the expert, the proper units are much larger, including familiar letter groupings, words and occasional phrases. Similarly, the beginning driver laboriously struggles to harmonise clutch, gas pedal, steering wheel, and brake, to the considerable terror of innocent bystanders. After a while, those movements come quite routinely and are subsumed under much higher (though perhaps equally dangerous) chunks of behaviour such as overtaking another car. (Gleitman, 1991)

Thus, 'much of the difference between master and apprentice is in the degree to which subcomponents of the activity have been chunked hierarchically' (Gleitman, 1991).

When applied to nursing, the chunks take the form of sets of procedures or groups of related past paradigm cases which the expert nurse calls on unconsciously, such that 'this multifaceted knowledge with its concrete referents cannot really be put into abstract principles or even explicit guidelines' and 'if experts are made to attend to the particulars or to a formal model or rule, their performance actually deteriorates' (Benner, 1984).

The idea that practitioners progress from conscious to unconscious knowledge has also been postulated in the field of teacher education, where Saville (cited in Schratz and Walker, 1995) described a learning sequence of:

From   unconscious incompetence
to   conscious incompetence
to   conscious competence
to   unconscious competence

These stages correspond, albeit loosely, to Benner's first four stages of novice, advanced beginner, competent and proficient nurse, and she would no doubt wish to add a fifth stage of unconscious expertise to Saville's sequence.

This notion of unconscious expertise has very clear advantages for activities which are based predominantly on motor skills, and which can be carried out automatically, such as driving and typing, and may even be of use to the nurse–technician who is concerned with the one-way process of applying theory to practice, since her theory acquisition occurs outside of the clinical setting, either by reading, by attending lectures, or by reflection-on-action.

However, Benner's model, which she borrowed from the work of Dreyfus and Dreyfus, is based on a view of expertise in all fields as essentially the same. In particular, Dreyfus and Dreyfus failed to distinguish between motor skill expertise and cognitive expertise, and intermingled examples of the expert driver, the expert pilot and the chess grandmaster. Arguably, however, motor skills and cognitive abilities are very different and expertise in each is arrived at by a different process. Thus, to talk of the expert driver and the expert chess player in the same way is to make what Ryle (1963) referred to as a category mistake.

With regard to motor skills, Dreyfus and Dreyfus are correct in the following observation:

> Have you ever been driving effortlessly along a city street in a stick-shift car and suddenly found yourself consciously thinking about the gear you are in and whether it's appropriate? Chances are the sudden reflection upon what you were doing and the rules for doing it was accompanied by a severe degradation of performance; perhaps you shifted at the wrong time or into the wrong gear. (Dreyfus and Dreyfus, 1986)

Motor skills rely on an interplay between brain, body and eye which circumvents rational cognition and, as most expert car drivers, pilots, pianists and typists will tell you, their performance deteriorates significantly when attended to.

However, cognitive abilities (I hesitate even to refer to them as skills) are of a different order, and whereas expertise in motor skills is acquired by repeated and mechanical practice, the expertise of the chess grandmaster is clearly not. As Dreyfus and Dreyfus themselves pointed out:

> Not all people achieve an expert level in their skills. Some areas of skill — chess, for example — have the characteristics that only a very small fraction of beginners can ever master the domain.... Other areas, such as automobile driving, are so designed that almost all novices can eventually reach the level we call expert. (Dreyfus and Dreyfus, 1986)

I would suggest that the difference between chess and driving is not merely quantitative as Dreyfus and Dreyfus seem to be suggesting, but qualitative. For the vast majority of people, no amount of practice will ever result in their becoming chess grandmasters because expertise in chess is not acquired in the same way as expertise in driving, but requires the player to process and store a vast number of past paradigm cases through active, conscious reflection on them.

Thus, while unconscious expertise is probably the highest stage of attainment for technical motor skills, cognitive abilities are somewhat different. Dreyfus and Dreyfus (1986) themselves recognised this when they asked the question: 'What does a masterful chess player think about when time permits, even when an intuitively obvious move has already come spontaneously to mind?'.

The answer, they tell us, is that she thinks about chess in a process of 'deliberative rationality', unlike the expert car driver who generally thinks about anything but driving. Of course, the chess grandmaster does not have to think about chess; she can, as Dreyfus and Dreyfus demonstrated in an experiment, do mental arithmetic, and her performance will not be significantly impaired. But the point is that thinking about chess will make her a better chess player in a way that thinking about typing will not make for a better typist.

In the same way, it is possible for an expert nurse to do mental arithmetic while nursing, but she will be a better nurse if she is thinking about what she is doing. Thus, for the nurse–practitioner who is concerned with reflection-in-action, with on-the-spot experimenting and with the generation of theory and the testing of hypotheses in the practice situation, it is vitally important that she is acutely conscious of the clinical situation she finds herself in, and this requires her to go beyond expertise as both Benner and Dreyfus and Dreyfus describe it.

Going beyond expertise, in one sense, involves the exact opposite of skilfulness, and will be referred to here as advanced practice. Whereas the aim of a skilled performance is to act intuitively and without conscious thought, almost at spinal cord level, the advanced nurse–practitioner requires a particular sort of mindfulness which involves an intense concentration on the task at hand. Even with very simple tasks such as wound dressing, the contrast is striking: the expert nurse–technician would perform the required actions swiftly and deftly and without conscious thought (and could even be doing mental arithmetic if she so desired!), whereas the advanced nurse-practitioner would think about every move, every decision, relating them to this patient in this situation. More importantly, she would be learning from her performance, thinking about how it could be done differently, constructing theories, testing hypotheses, and modifying her actions in the here and now, and this requires mindful attention. A description of this approach to advanced nursing practice is provided in Part 2 of this book.

This active, mindful, continuous learning process is in direct contrast to the skilled performance of the expert, for whom:

> as a practice becomes more repetitive and routine, and as knowing-in-practice becomes increasingly tacit and spontaneous, the practitioner may miss important opportunities to think about what he is doing. He may find that... he is drawn into patterns of error which he cannot correct. And if he learns, as often happens, to be selectively inattentive to phenomena that do not fit the categories of his knowing-in-action, then he may suffer from boredom or 'burn out' and afflict his clients with the consequences of his narrowness and rigidity. When this happens, the practitioner has 'over-learned' what he knows. (Schön, 1983)

Reflection-in-action therefore serves to focus the attention of the nurse-practitioner on the here-and-now and on the uniqueness of her individual relationships with each of her patients, and reduces the possibility of the boredom and burn out that comes from overfamiliarity with the tasks to be performed. Thus, we can add a sixth stage to Saville's learning sequence, as shown in Table 3.1.

Educating the advanced nurse–practitioner

The difference between the expert nurse-technician and the advanced nurse-practitioner is therefore in the final link from practice back to informal theory as shown in Figure 3.2f. Whereas expertise as defined above is the most appropriate process for the smooth and effective translation of theory into practice, it is of limited use in reflexively generating theory back out of practice, which requires the practitioner to act in a mindful way. Education for the advanced nurse-practitioner is therefore not concerned with the development of skills and

Table 3.1 A sequence of learning

Saville	Benner
unconscious incompetence	novice
conscious incompetence	advanced beginner
conscious competence	competent
unconscious competence	proficient
(unconscious expertise)	expert
(conscious expertise)	(advanced)

expertise, but with fostering reflection-in-action and mindful practice, with moving from unconscious expertise to conscious expertise.

A course for advanced nursing practice should begin with three assumptions: firstly, that the nurse–practitioner has already mastered reflection-on-action, and is employing it as a regular part of her practice; secondly, that she has learnt how to gain access to formal theory and public knowledge, and is doing so as a regular part of her practice; and thirdly, that she is an expert in her own clinical specialism with a well-developed knowledge and skills base. The relationship between the nurse–practitioner and the teacher is one of equals, of experts in their own particular fields of practice and education respectively; the teacher does not presume to impart any formal theory or knowledge to the practitioner, but acts as a facilitator. The course is therefore content-free in that no external material is introduced by the facilitator of learning. Rather, practitioner and facilitator work together on the practitioner's informal theory and personal knowledge, using critical incident analysis and clinical supervision techniques, focusing particularly on reflection-in-action, on the interplay between practice and informal theory. This is not inconsistent with the UKCC's proposals for education of the Advanced Practitioner, which is concerned with:

> adjusting the boundaries for the development of future practice, pioneering and developing new roles responsive to changing needs and with advancing clinical practice, research and education in order to enrich professional practice as a whole. (UKCC, 1990)

Such a course would therefore be practice-focused, but not skills-based. It would be concerned with turning experience into informal theory, and informal theory into action in a seamless, integrated process. It would be concerned with developing on-the-spot researching and on-the-spot decision making, with becoming an autonomous practitioner in the true sense of the word, being able to generate one's own theory, carry out one's own research and justify one's clinical decisions from informal as well as from formal theory.

Because the course would focus on process rather than on content, it would be appropriate to bring together practitioners from different specialisms, and even from different disciplines, and because the cognitive skills required would be of a very high order, such a course should be at least at Masters' level, if not higher. Again, this is consistent with UKCC recommendations. However, it would not be a traditional taught Masters degree, but would more closely resemble a Master of Philosophy (MPhil) course, where each individual student would be pursuing his own learning in relation to his clinical specialism, closely supervised by an advanced nurse–practitioner and an educationalist. But unlike traditional MPhil degrees, which are research-based, this would be a Masters degree by practice, which would be examined by a substantial piece of written work focusing on a particular practice issue. This would include the student's reflection-on-action, accounts and analyses of his reflection-in-action, and would integrate his personal knowledge and informal theory with public knowledge and formal theory.

References

Abercrombie, M.L.J. (1979) *Aims and Techniques of Group Teaching*. Guildford: SRHE.

Benner, P. (1984) *From Novice to Expert*. California: Addison-Wesley.

Bines, H. (1992) Issues in course design. In: *Developing Professional Education* (H. Bines and D. Watson, eds) Buckingham: Open University Press.

Boud, D., Keogh, R. and Walker, D. (1985) *Reflection: Turning Experience into Learning*. London: Kogan Page.

Boyd, E.M. and Fales, A.W. (1983) Reflecting learning: key to learning from experience. *Journal of Humanistic Psychology*, **23**, 2, 99–117.

Brunner, J.S. (1966) *Towards a Theory of Instruction*. New York: Norton.

Champion, R. (1992) The philosophy of an honours degree programme in nursing and midwifery. In: *Developing Professional Education* (H. Bines and D. Watson, eds) Buckingham: Open University Press.

Dewey, J. (1916) *Democracy and Education*. New York: The Free Press.

Dreyfus, H.L. and Dreyfus, S.E. (1977) Uses and abuses of multiattribute and multi-aspect model of decision making. Unpublished manuscript cited in Benner (1984) *From Novice to Expert*. California: Addison-Wesley.

Dreyfus, H.L. and Dreyfus, S.E. (1986) *Mind over Machine*. Oxford: Blackwell.

ENB (1990) *Devolved Continuous Assessment for Courses leading to Parts 1, 3, 5, 8, 12, 13, 14 and 15 of the Professional Register*. London: ENB.

Fitzgerald, M. (1994) Theories of reflection for learning. In: *Reflective Practice in Nursing*, (A. Palmer, S. Burns and C. Bulman, eds) Oxford: Blackwell Scientific.

Gibbs, G. (1992) *Improving the Quality of Student Learning*. Bristol: Technical and Educational Services.

Glazer, N. (1974) Schools of the minor professions *Minerva*, **12** (13) 346-363.

Gleitman, H. (1991) *Psychology*. New York: Norton.

Jasper, M. and Rolfe, G. (1993) A framework for a process-driven Common Foundation Programme for graduates. *International Journal of Nursing Studies*, **30**, 5, 377-385.

Kolb, D.A. and Fry, R. (1975) Towards an applied theory of experiential learning. In: *The Theories of Group Processes* (C.L. Cooper, ed.) London: John Lilley and Sons.

Lawton, D. (1980) *The Politics of the School Curriculum*. London: Routledge and Kegan Paul.

Maddox, H. (1963) *How to Study*. London: Pan.

McNiff, J. (1993) *Teaching as Learning*. London: Routledge.

Reed, J. and Procter, S. (1993) *Nurse Education: A Reflective Approach*. London: Edward Arnold.

Rogers, C.R. (1957) Personal thoughts on teaching and learning. *Merrill-Palmer Quarterly*, **3**, 241-243.

Rogers, C.R. (1969) *Freedom to Learn: A View of what Education might Become*. Columbus: Charles E. Merrill.

Rogers, C. (1983) *Freedom to Learn for the 80s*. Ohio: Merrill.

Rolfe, G. and Jasper, M. (1993) Some strategies for curriculum development in nurse education. *Journal of Further and Higher Education*, **17**, 3, 105-111.

Ryle, G. (1963) *The Concept of Mind*. Harmondsworth: Penguin.

Schein, E. (1973) *Professional Education*. New York: McGraw-Hill.

Schön, D.A. (1983) *The Reflective Practitioner*. London: Temple Smith.

Schön, D.A. (1987) *Educating the Reflective Practitioner*. San Francisco: Jossey-Bass.

Schratz, M. and Walker, R. (1995) *Research as Social Change*. London: Routledge.

UKCC (1990) *The Report of the Post-Graduate Practice Project*. London: UKCC.

4

Towards a new paradigm for nursing

Probably the single most prevalent claim advanced by the proponents of a new paradigm is that they can solve the problems that have led the old one to a crisis.

Thomas Kuhn

I must create my own System or be enslaved by another man's.
My business is not to reason and compare;
my business is to create.

William Blake

Nursing in crisis

The problem of the theory-practice gap is the most important, and at the same time, the most fundamental issue currently facing nursing, since if the profession cannot be certain that theory is being reliably and accurately translated into good nursing practice, then it cannot be certain of anything. It has been argued in the preceding chapters that the continued presence of the theory-practice gap is a symptom of a major crisis for the nursing profession, namely that the existing scientific paradigm of technical rationality on which nursing is built is no longer adequate to meet the needs of practising nurses.

It has been shown that the technical rationality paradigm is particularly suited to disciplines which take a macro approach, where, by its very nature, it results in an almost perfect match between theory and practice in both the 'hard' and the 'soft' sciences. Two arguments have been put forward in this book as to why the match between theory and practice is so close, and they will be very briefly recapped here.

Firstly, the technical rationality paradigm, *by its very nature*, is designed to minimise the theory-practice gap. Altrichter *et al.* (1993) have summarised the main tenets of technical rationality as:

- there are general solutions to practical problems;
- these solutions can be developed outside practical situations (in research or administrative centres);
- the solutions can be translated into practitioners' actions by means of publications, training, administrative orders, etc.

It can be clearly seen that, if adhered to, these tenets provide for a smooth translation from researchers' findings into practitioners' actions through the application of general solutions to universal problems, and that theoretically at least, we should not expect there to be a gap between what is postulated in theory and what actually works in practice. The price to be paid for this, however, is a hierarchical split between the scientists who do the thinking and the technicians who implement the scientists' theories.

The second argument advanced in this book is that we know simply by looking around us that the technical rationality paradigm is effective. It is almost universally acknowledged that science and technology have been spectacularly successful in transforming the world, in most technical disciplines there are very few problems in translating research findings into practical applications. For example, in civil engineering the gap between theory and practice is so small as to be almost non-existent, and if a bridge is designed to carry a specific load in theory, then it will almost certainly carry that load in practice.

The fact that the theory-practice gap is so prominent in nursing is therefore an indication that the technical rationality paradigm is inappropriate for current practice, which is increasingly taking a micro, individual approach to nursing care. This is an embarrassment to those nurse academics and researchers who wish to promote nursing as a technical science, and in their attempt to minimise the significance of the gap, they have tried to portray it as a minor irritation, largely the fault of practitioners who are unable to put theory into practice, or even to totally ignore it in the hope that it will go away.

So why is the gap so great in nursing compared to other disciplines? Kuhn (1962) suggested that the evolution of science is cyclical. Periods of what he referred to as 'normal science', when current theory and knowledge appear to provide answers to the problems of the day, give way to periods of crisis, when questions begin to be asked about the adequacy of science to account for happenings in the real world. It is in periods of crisis that the gap between theory and practice becomes apparent, and bridges start to fall down!

Finally, crisis gives way to revolution, to shifts and changes in the current paradigm, and a new period of normal science is established. However, during periods of crisis, proponents of normal science will do their utmost to deny or minimise the problems, and to blame the fallen bridges on the builders, preferring the security of the old to the challenge of the new. For example, in the sixteenth century, church leaders who upheld the geocentric model of the universe condemned their opponents to death as heretics rather than accept the growing evidence that the Earth revolved around the Sun rather than *vice versa*.

Similarly, from the 'normal science' perspective of the current nursing paradigm, not only is the theory–practice gap not recognised as a crisis, it is not even acknowledged as a problem, although thankfully we have abolished the death penalty for those who disagree. As Kuhn pointed out:

> One of the things a scientific community acquires with a paradigm is a criterion for choosing problems that, while the paradigm is taken for granted, can be assumed to have solutions. To a great extent, these are the only problems that the community will admit as scientific or encourage its members to undertake. (Kuhn, 1962)

The community of nursing academics, then, has chosen either consciously or unconsciously not to define the theory–practice gap as a problem to be explored, since to do so would be to admit that the gap is not entirely the result of bad or inadequate practice, but rather that nursing is in a period of crisis, and that perhaps theory, and the way in which it is generated and disseminated, is at least partly to blame.

In the preceding chapters, an attempt was made to demonstrate that the current, albeit largely unacknowledged, crisis is the result of an incompatibility between nursing practice on the one hand, and nursing theory, education and research on the other. It was argued that whereas nursing practice has moved 'from the established pattern of practice based on routinisation, allocation of tasks, and adherence to management and medical models' (Pearson, 1988) towards a patient-centred, holistic, humanistic approach based on interpersonal therapeutic relationships; nursing theory, and the way that theory is generated and disseminated, has not kept apace. It is as though there has been a radical shift in the way that engineers construct bridges, although the designers are still drawing up plans based on the old, outdated methods.

Nursing in revolution

There are two possible solutions to the current crisis in nursing. Firstly, practice could shift back into line with theory, that is, nurses could return to a more technical approach to nursing care, to caring for rather than caring about their patients. As nursing practice once more became a technical issue of logistics, of the management of patients and tasks, then the global, macro, statistical nature of nursing knowledge and theory, generated through the traditional scientific research paradigm, would again address and answer the relevant questions for practice. The crisis would be averted and the discipline of nursing would revert back to normal science.

Secondly, theory could move into line with current philosophies of practice. Concepts of what nursing theory and knowledge is, how it is generated, and how it is passed on, could be reformulated to meet the demands of what is essentially an interpersonal, humanistic discipline requiring a micro, individualised approach to knowledge and theory. The period of crisis would give way to revolution, and eventually to a new period of normal science, built on a new theoretical foundation; in other words, there would be what Kuhn referred to as a paradigm shift.

This second option of a paradigm shift and a revolution in nursing theory is the one that has been pursued in this book. Chapter 1 argued for a new conception of knowledge and theory, based on a modified version of the scientific method referred to as hypothetico-abductivism, in which individual cases are employed to inform other individual cases. A model of nursing praxis, the coming together of theory and practice, was constructed, drawing on Donald Schön's notions of reflection-on-action and reflection-in-action, and a contrast was made between the nurse–technician, who adheres to the traditional technical rationality paradigm of nursing, and the nurse–practitioner, who employs the model of nursing praxis and who generates her own informal theory and personal knowledge out of her own practice.

Chapter 2 began by claiming that the traditional scientific research paradigm has little to offer the nurse–practitioner, whose practice is grounded in the interpersonal relationships she has with her patients. It was argued that a new model of nursing research, which operates on an individual micro level rather than on a generalisable macro level, is required; a model which generates theory of direct relevance to individual encounters between the nurse and her patients, and which closes the theory–practice gap by directly bringing about clinical change. Notions of reflective and reflexive research were introduced, and were combined with traditional scientific research approaches into a new model of practitioner-based research for nursing praxis. This model was expounded at length, and the problems of implementing it within the current research climate were explored.

Chapter 3 examined the role of education in nursing praxis, and noted that recent developments such as the introduction of the Project 2000 curriculum and the move of nurse education into the university sector reflect the continued support given to the technical rationality paradigm, and conform to what Bines described as the technocratic model of education. In contrast, it was argued that the nurse–practitioner has very different educational needs; in particular, she is concerned with the generation of her own personal knowledge and informal theory, for which technocratic education makes no provision. A post-technocratic model was proposed, which has a number of profound implications for nurse education. A philosophy of teaching and learning relevant to post-technocratic education was also described, and a curriculum framework for initial nurse training based on a reflective spiral was suggested. Finally, the model was extended to the educational needs of qualified nurses, and suggestions were made for education for expertise and beyond.

Very few of the ideas and theories presented in the preceding chapters are new. Informal theory, although not often formally acknowledged in nursing, formed the basis of Benner's conception of the expert nurse, and nursing recognised the importance of reflective practice some years ago, and it now features in many nursing curricula. In research, the small-scale, micro approach borrows heavily from the educational models of practitioner-based enquiry, action research and new paradigm research. And in education, the philosophy of student-centred learning dates back at least 40 years, and possibly back to Rousseau in the eighteenth century, while Jerome Bruner introduced the concept of the spiral curriculum in the 1960s.

What *is* new about these ideas and theories is the way in which they have been brought together and integrated into holistic models of theory, research and education which are congruent with current approaches to nursing practice. Furthermore, if a paradigm consists of 'law, theory, applications and instrumentation together' (Kuhn, 1962), then the model of nursing praxis, the model of practitioner-based research, and the model of post-technocratic education taken together and underpinned by the scientific process of hypothetico-abductivism, constitutes a new paradigm for nursing (Figure 4.1).

This new paradigm is based on what Altrichter *et al.* referred to as reflective rationality. In contrast to the tenets of technical rationality outlined at the beginning of this chapter, reflective rationality is based on the assumptions that:

- complex practical problems demand specific solutions;
- these solutions can be developed only inside the context in which the problem arises and in which the practitioner is a crucial and determining element;
- the solutions cannot be successfully applied to other contexts but they can be made accessible to other practitioners as hypotheses to be tested.

(Altrichter *et al.*, 1993)

The basis of the new paradigm is the model of nursing praxis, the coming together of theory and practice as an integrated whole. Praxis involves both reflective and reflexive practice. Reflective practice is inward looking and is the foundation on

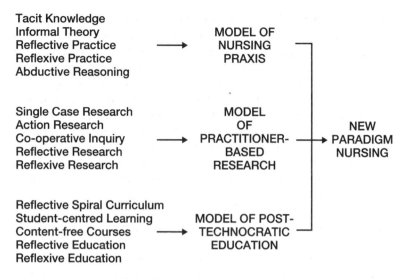

Figure 4.1 A new paradigm for nursing

which the new paradigm is built; it involves detailed self-examination either through diary writing or in clinical supervision. Through consideration of her own practice, the nurse–practitioner generates personal knowledge, and through analysis of that knowledge, she transforms it into informal theory. In doing reflective practice, the nurse–practitioner therefore also becomes involved in her own research and education.

In contrast, reflexive practice is at a more advanced level and requires the nurse to think on her feet rather than in the luxury of supervision. It is outward looking, and is concerned with bringing about clinical change. Reflexive practice involves on-the-spot experimenting and theory construction, and is a form of research and education in action, unlike reflective practice which is conducted away from the clinical setting and after the event. True reflexive practice is a rare thing in nursing, simply because the profession does not recognise it as a component of advanced practice, and therefore nurses are rarely trained in it. However, techniques borrowed from family therapy such as hypothesising and live supervision come close to being reflexive practice, and will be explored more fully in Part 2 of this book.

Thus, although the three areas of theory, research and education have been addressed in separate chapters, the new paradigm integrates them fully. To practice is to research and to learn, since reflective and reflexive practice both involve the generation and transformation of personal knowledge into informal theory, so that it is impossible to be a new paradigm nurse–practitioner without also becoming involved in researching one's own practice and in one's own education. Theory, practice, research and education therefore merge into the single, indivisible whole of nursing praxis.

Towards a new paradigm

Models, theories and maps

It could be argued, of course, that the new paradigm merely replaces old models with new ones. In order to respond to this criticism that nursing praxis is merely old medicine in new bottles, it is necessary to examine precisely what the nursing profession understands by a model, a task which is complicated by 'the vague terminology used and the lack of clear interrelationships between concepts' (Manley, 1991). General definitions of models in nursing often refer to:

> a graphic and symbolic representation of a phenomenon that serves to objectify and present a certain perspective or point of view about its nature and/or function. (Powers and Knapp, 1990)

Models, then, are representations of objects, properties or events from the real world. Models can be made of physical material, they can be diagrams, they can be mathematical formulas, or they can be words. Physical models are the most commonly encountered in everyday life, and can sometimes be perfect replicas, retaining all the detail of the original, but more usually they are simplifications or analogues. A simplified model aids understanding by omitting confusing or irrelevant elements, as, for example, in an architect's model for a new house. An analogue model aids understanding by substituting a known and intelligible phenomenon for an unknown and unintelligible one, for example, in attempting to understand the workings of an atom by representing it as a miniature solar system.

When we talk about models of nursing, however, we are usually referring to something rather different from physical models. As Robinson (1993) pointed out:

> Nurses may indeed use scale models, such as those of the heart or kidney, in order to learn about the structure and function of the human body, but these are emphatically *not* nursing models.

Nursing models, in contrast, are usually either conceptual or theoretical, that is, 'they identify concepts and describe their relationships to the phenomena of central concern to the discipline' (Powers and Knapp, 1990). These 'phenomena of central concern' almost always include the person/patient, the environment, health, and nursing (Fawcett, 1984), and because most models are concerned with such global concepts, they are often referred to as grand theories (Chinn and Jacobs, 1987).

This close association between models and theories is recognised by most nurse academics, although the exact nature of the relationship can be somewhat confusing. It is generally agreed, however, that *conceptual* models are used in conjunction with theory in order to build, illustrate or supplement it, whereas *theoretical* models, as their name suggests, are virtually synonymous with theory, and represent a written theory in some other form, usually pictorial or diagrammatic. Thus, 'theorists often move back and forth between expressing theories in written sentences and visual devices, such as diagrams, during theory construction' (Walker and Avant, 1988). To confuse matters even further, some writers use the terms 'model' and 'theory' almost interchangeably. Chinn and Kramer (1991), for example, claimed that 'for us, conceptual and theoretic models coexist with theory', while Meleis (1985) suggested that the difference between models and theories is more semantic than substantive, and that 'the final choice of a label is a personal matter and depends on the purpose for which the label is applied'.

It has been argued throughout Part 1 of this book that generalisable, scientific, formal theory is only of secondary importance to the nurse–practitioner, who is more concerned with personal knowledge and informal theory generated from her own clinical experiences through reflection-on-action. But if there is no real difference between a formal theory and a model, what use does the nurse-practitioner have for the models of praxis, of research and of education presented in this book?

In order to answer that question, it is necessary to compare these models with the traditional nursing models discussed previously. Whereas the function of traditional models is to build, illustrate, support or conceptualise formal, generalisable theory, the function of the models of praxis, research and education outlined in this book is to build, illustrate, support and conceptualise *informal*, personal theory. But while traditional formal models have been described as standing for or representing formal theory, clearly this is not possible in the case of informal models, since informal theory, by definition, is fluctuating, dynamic, and unique to each and every practitioner. There is no identifiable body of informal theory which relates to nursing as a whole, and therefore no single model that can represent every practitioner's unique and different body of informal theory. The relationship between informal models and informal theories is therefore very different from that between formal models and formal theories, and goes beyond simple concrete representation.

But if informal models cannot represent, illustrate or conceptualise the *content* of informal theories, what then do they represent? The answer, which can be seen by examining the informal models presented in this book, is that they represent the *process* of constructing informal theory. Whereas formal models help us to understand the content of formal, generalisable theory which can then be applied to practice, informal models help us to understand how we can construct our own informal, personal theory out of practice. Thus, while the formal models contribute to the separation of theory and practice, informal models help to unite them.

Informal models are therefore process models, in that they describe how theory can be generated rather than saying anything about the theory itself. They are content-free, and as such, bear more similarity to maps than they do to models: whereas a model is concerned with representation, a map is concerned with orientation. Models are useful for representing, conceptualising and simplifying the world. They tell you 'what' rather than 'how', and are useful in theory building, and in disciplines where theory building is the main concern, such as sociology. Maps, on the other hand, are useful for finding your way around; they show you where you are in relation to where you want to be. They tell you 'how' rather than 'what', and are useful in practice development and in disciplines where practice is the main concern, such as nursing. Furthermore, maps involve us in a creative process, since as Ziman (1978) pointed out, 'more information can be read from a map than was needed to construct it'.

As an example, let us compare Roper, Logan and Tierney's 'Activities of Daily Living' (ADL) model with the informal model of nursing praxis outlined in this book. The model of praxis stands in the same relation to the ADL model as does a map to a set of directions. A set of directions will tell you how to get from where you are to where you want to be, for example, by taking the first left, second right, etc., whereas a map will merely *show* you where you are in relation to where you want to be. Unlike a set of directions, it will not prescribe a route. How you get from A to B is up to you; there might be several routes, and you must choose which is the best one for you. Formal models such as the ADL are therefore most appropriate for the nurse–technician since they provide a set of guidelines for practice. Informal, process models such as the model of praxis, on the other hand, are most appropriate for the nurse–practitioner, since they allow her to make individual decisions based on her own body of informal theory and personal knowledge in each new situation.

Problems in establishing a new paradigm

It is being argued that the models outlined in this book together form the basis for a new paradigm. Powers and Knapp (1990) claimed that a paradigm is an organising framework which contains:

- concepts, theories, assumptions, beliefs, values and principles that form a way for a discipline to interpret the subject matter with which it is concerned;
- research methods considered to be best suited to generating knowledge within this frame of reference;
- what is open to investigation — priorities and views on knowledge deficit areas where research and theory building is most needed;
- what is closed to inquiry for a time.

It can be seen from this list that the dominant paradigm exerts a great deal of influence over the direction that a profession or discipline takes. Not only does the paradigm define what counts as knowledge, how that knowledge is generated and how it is disseminated, but also the assumptions, beliefs, values and principles underpinning that knowledge. Furthermore, adherence to the accepted rules and methods of the paradigm is a way of ensuring exclusivity within the profession, such that:

> By placing a heavy emphasis on correct method, all members of a scientific community are assured a kind of collective protection: madmen, charlatans, fakers, and sophists are hopefully excluded from the ranks. (Phillips, 1973)

Whoever exerts influence and control over the dominant paradigm therefore wields considerable power, and in the nursing profession, the power to define the rules and values of the discipline is vested in a small elite of teachers, researchers and academics.

The problem of scientism

As might be expected, challenges to this academic elite are extremely difficult, since any meaningful change is actively discouraged by placing ever tighter constraints on what legitimately counts as practice, research and education. For practitioners, pressure to engage in practice based exclusively on the findings from traditional scientific research is so great that anyone questioning the validity of this approach to informing practice is looked upon with great suspicion and is regarded as outdated and even as dangerous, as though practice is either informed by technical, scientific research or it is not informed at all.

Sayer (1992) referred to this attitude as scientism, 'the striking tendency... to assume that [traditional] science is the highest form of knowledge, to which all should aspire'. Like sexism or racism, scientism is the unjustified imposition of a particular viewpoint to the exclusion of others; a sort of methodological hegemony. Hollis described the mechanisms through which scientism works:

Normal science is... kept on track by social mechanisms. It is highly organised activity, usually with a hierarchical power structure. Young scientists serve apprenticeships, in which they learn to think and practise as required by the prevailing paradigm, and they are promoted for learning the lesson well. The heroic saga of the isolated individual genius is purely a myth. Real scientists work in hierarchical communities, subject to a discipline which reinforces the paradigm. Also they need funds. Science is an industry with investors to satisfy as well as an exercise in curiosity. That usually means pleasing the government, whose aims are not disinterested. Those who pay the piper call the tune. Thus the knowledge industry is enmeshed in a wider social and political system, which helps further to explain why a particular paradigm persists and how it regulates the practice of science. (Hollis, 1994)

In nursing research, the technical, hard science, medical model paradigm is strengthening its hold, particularly since the publication of the *Report of the Taskforce on the Strategy for Research in Nursing, Midwifery and Health Visiting* on behalf of the Government in 1993, to the point that it is now almost impossible to obtain major funding for research projects that are not carried out by multidisciplinary teams and that do not employ large samples to produce generalisable findings. Clearly, that approach to research has its place, but this book has argued that there is also a place for research which is concerned specifically and exclusively with nursing issues, which is carried out by practising nurses with their own patients in their own workplace, and which might not be generalisable far beyond those nurses and patients and that workplace.

However, this practitioner-based approach to reflective and reflexive research is specifically excluded from the concept of nursing research offered by the Taskforce, which defined it as 'rigorous and systematic enquiry... designed to lead to generalisable contributions to knowledge' in which 'small scale projects should be curbed' (Department of Health, 1993). The new paradigm researcher is therefore forced to go it alone, without funding and without formal recognition, at least from her own profession.

And in nurse education, the introduction of the Project 2000 curriculum and the move into higher education are reinforcing the grip of the technocratic model on the training and education of nurses and the domination of formal, scientific theory over practice. New, innovative curriculum models are becoming increasingly difficult to introduce, not necessarily because the professional governing bodies are opposed to innovation in education, but because of the practical problems of teaching large classes and of meeting the rather technical outcomes required by most nursing syllabuses.

The problem of the shift in power

As if these were not obstacles enough, in the case of the new paradigm outlined in this book there are added problems. Not only does the new paradigm involve a radical shift in understanding and defining what knowledge is, how it is generated and how it is transmitted, but it also involves a shift in the power base itself, from a small group of researchers, educators and academics to the profession as a whole. In the new paradigm, it is practitioners who define what knowledge is, who determine the relative value attached to different types of knowledge, who specify the problems for research, who carry out the research, who own the research findings, and who control the dissemination of knowledge through the education process. We should therefore expect enormous resistance to any paradigm where power is shifted from the hands of the few to the hands of the many.

The problem of communicating across paradigms

The above problem is compounded by the fact that the existing paradigm is now so established that any new paradigm will inevitably be judged according to the values, beliefs and methodological rules of the old. Even communication across paradigms is difficult. Darbyshire (1994) pointed out that when a world view 'notable for its emphasis on the laudability of formal systems, rules, universally accepted definitions, measurement, objective validation, empirical testing, falsifying hypotheses and so on' is so pervasive, 'suggesting an alternative to this entire schema of what counts as knowledge... can be like trying to dialogue with Daleks'.

The extent of this communication problem is demonstrated by the criteria outlined by David Hume in the nineteenth century for judging the worth of an academic work:

> If we take in our hand any volume; of divinity or school metaphysics, for instance; let us ask, Does it contain any abstract reasoning concerning quantity or number? No. Does it contain any experimental reasoning concerning matter of fact and existence? No. Commit it then to the flames: for it can contain nothing but sophistry and illusion. (Hume, 1875)

Hume was an empiricist philosopher who believed that knowledge could only be obtained through the senses, apart from certain a priori truths such as those expressed by mathematics. If a book contained no mathematical reasoning and no experimental studies, then by definition, it contained no knowledge and should be rejected out of hand, whatever its subject matter. Challenges to the empiricist view of the world which came from a non-empiricist position were therefore seen as 'sophistry and illusion', and consigned, unread, to the flames.

Clearly, there has been some progress over the centuries, from the burning of dissenters in the time of Copernicus to the burning of their books in the time of Hume (although the case of Salman Rushdie might be seen as an exception). At least these days critics usually read the books before they burn them, but the problem still remains that any alternatives to the dominant paradigm will inevitably be judged according to the values and academic rules of that paradigm.

Thus, critics of this new paradigm, judging it from the perspective of the established 'normal science', will inevitably point out the lack of academic rigour applied to the generation of informal theory, they will question the status of personal, tacit knowledge as 'real' knowledge, they will criticise the model of research for its lack of methodological rigour and its overtly subjective stance, and they will criticise the model of education for its lack of externally imposed syllabus material and point out the dangers of allowing students to identify and meet their own learning needs. However, as Bateson (1979) observed, 'the division of the perceived universe into parts and wholes is convenient and may be necessary, but no necessity determines how it shall be done', and to paraphrase Darbyshire, criticising the new paradigm for not meeting the standards of the old paradigm is rather like criticising a car for being a bad bicycle.

The problem of resistance to a questioning attitude

A further reason for possible resistance to this new paradigm lies in its reflective nature. Methods of enquiry which are inward looking and self-critical generally pose far more of a threat to the status quo than those which look outwards, and tend to be rejected with far more vigour. As the philosopher Bernard Williams (1985) noted, 'reflection can destroy knowledge'. By this, he did not mean that reflection was a destructive force, but that it can introduce uncertainty into a hitherto unquestioned world view, and that 'people's sense of social and moral direction can depend on not asking too many questions' (Hollis, 1994). Reflective practitioners are therefore often perceived as trouble makers, out to upset the applecart.

The problem of immature science

There is yet another criticism of *any* new paradigm in nursing which must be addressed, and that is the argument that paradigm shifts are impossible since it is not appropriate to regard nursing as possessing a paradigm at all. Robinson (1993), for example, has claimed that nursing is not yet a mature science and thus cannot be said to operate from within a paradigm as defined by Kuhn. She went on to contrast mature sciences such as physics, which possess 'a strong sense of commonality', with nursing, which she claimed has unclear boundaries, problems which are loosely defined, an unspecific theoretical structure, and a concern with a qualitative pattern of enquiry.

However, disputes about the level of maturity of nursing are rather spurious, since the notion that only mature sciences can lay claim to paradigms is a circular argument at best, and tautologous at worst. If, firstly, the paradigm of a scientific community comprises a shared set of laws, theories, applications and instrumentations which are 'revealed in its textbooks, lectures, and laboratory exercises' (Kuhn, 1962), and if, secondly, a mature science is one which displays a strong sense of commonality, then a shared paradigm clearly contributes to the maturity of a scientific community, and a mature science is therefore to some extent defined by the paradigm it operates within. To argue that nursing cannot posses a paradigm because it is not yet a mature science misses the point that one of the steps to becoming a mature science with a strong consensus of opinion is the adoption of a shared paradigm. At some point, then, an immature discipline such as nursing must agree on a shared paradigm as a step towards maturity.

Furthermore, I would disagree with Robinson's assessment of nursing as being unfocused and lacking a world view, and indeed with her assertion that it lacks a shared paradigm. Nursing has defined itself as a social activity, and, it has been argued in previous chapters, has adopted the paradigm of the social sciences. Whether this is the best or the most appropriate paradigm is another matter entirely, and a disagreement over boundaries and theoretical structure might, as Robinson suggests, indicate immaturity, but it might also indicate a growing dissatisfaction with the dominant paradigm. In any case, Kuhn employed the term 'paradigm' in such a loose way that almost any discipline can be said to operate within one.

The problem of traditionalism

The final objection to the new paradigm to be considered here is the argument that the interpersonal relationship between nurse and patient is not after all the foundation of nursing. It has been assumed throughout this book that nursing practice has moved from being task oriented to person-centred, but there has recently been something of a backlash against this view, with a number of theorists calling for a return to the 'old values' of the traditional biomedical approach. This is clearly a potentially very damaging critique which needs to be dealt with at some length. The current state of the debate can be conveniently illustrated by examining three papers all from the same recent issue of the *Journal of Clinical Nursing* from March 1995.

In the guest editorial to celebrate 25 years of primary nursing, Barbara Vaughan advocated for an interpersonal focus based firmly on the nurse–patient relationship, claiming that:

> If nursing is routine and task based then the special contribution which can be made on the road to wellness... will be lost. Yet if the opportunity for personalised services, tailored for each recipient, is enhanced through an approach to care giving which facilitates a feeling of warmth and responsibility, then the true value of nursing can be realized. (Vaughan, 1995)

Interestingly, while Vaughan invokes the Patients' Charter and the emerging users' movement to support the cause of primary nursing, her opponents do likewise. In the same issue in which Vaughan's celebration of the silver anniversary of primary nursing appeared, so too did a paper entitled 'What are nurses doing to patients?', in which Ann Bradshaw mounted an eloquent plea for a return to a traditional approach to nursing based on routines, procedures and techniques underpinned by a mixture of biomedical science and common sense. Bradshaw looked back nostalgically to the 1960s when the emphasis of the nursing curriculum 'was very much on technical and practical procedures of physical care', and:

> great emphasis was placed on the correct way of bed making, bed bathing, aseptic dressing techniques, methods of relieving pressure, care of the unconscious patient, the administration of oxygen and last offices. (Bradshaw, 1995)

One of the main thrusts of her argument was that the so-called 'new nursing' movement has developed against the wishes of patients, whose overriding need is for 'excellent physical care' and a nurse–patient relationship based on nursing as a moral duty 'which maintains the necessity and inherent strength of a professional detachment within a bond of commitment and understanding' (Bradshaw, 1995).

In order to support her assertion that this is what patients really want, she firstly quoted from the novelist Alice Thomas Ellis, complaining in the *Daily Mail* about standards of cleanliness, care and discipline. What hospitals need, asserted Thomas Ellis, is 'a dose of common sense'. For Bradshaw, the fact that patients wish for a return to the traditional nursing model based on scientific medical knowledge is 'self-evident, a simple but universal truth for all people everywhere and from whatever culture', such that 'if we have been patients... we find ourselves murmuring our agreement'. I am not entirely sure that this 'evidence' is itself scientific medical knowledge, but Bradshaw did at least try to back up this 'simple but universal truth' by reference to a number of empirical research studies.

So what does the empirical research say? Fortunately, in the same issue of the *Journal of Clinical Nursing* is just such an empirical study by Christine Webb and Kevin Hope, entitled 'What kind of nurses do patients want?'. Webb and Hope also invoked the consumers' movement as justification for their study, and attempted to answer the question of what kind of nurses patients want by carrying out structured interviews with 103 patients, who were asked to rank order 12 activities chosen by the researchers as representative of the nurse's role.

Somewhat to the researchers' surprise, and in contrast to the findings from other studies cited in the literature review, 'the psychosocial aspects of listening to patients' worries and teaching them about their conditions receive the highest overall rankings'. Furthermore, 'relieving pain is the only physical/technical activity to achieve comparable ratings, but this too is an activity with strong emotional overtones' (Webb and Hope, 1995).

So what are we to conclude? Is it, as Bradshaw argued, a self-evident universal truth that patients desire a return to a traditional, technical, biomedical model of nursing based on professional detachment, in which case the entire foundation of this book begins to crumble. Or should we take heart from the findings of Webb and Hope that patients rank the psychosocial activities of nurses as most important? And are the activities of excellent physical care and psychosocial relationship building really as incompatible as Bradshaw seemed to imply when she claimed that 'the hard facts and techniques of rational experimental science are discredited and down-graded in favour of the narrative experiences of the intuitive caring relationship' (Bradshaw, 1995).

Having devoted a great deal of this book to the argument for why empirical research studies such as that reported here by Webb and Hope are of little value to nursing care, I can hardly now cite their work in defence of my thesis. However, a closer look at their findings will, I believe, illustrate not only why such studies are of little use to the nurse–practitioner, but also, ironically, why their general findings and conclusions are correct in spite of their methodology.

Webb and Hope found that the activity of listening to patients was ranked as most important by the greatest number of patients (24.5 per cent), with 53.1 per cent of all patients ranking it in the top three activities, and 8.7 per cent of patients believing that it is not a nursing duty at all. The most interesting thing about these data is not the percentage who thought that listening to patients is important, but the 46.9 per cent of patients who did not rank it in their top three activities at all. Thus, although listening to patients was ranked by patients themselves as the most important nursing activity, nearly half of those questioned did not include it in their top three, and a sizeable minority specifically considered it to be outside the scope of nursing.

These results illustrate perfectly my argument for the limited usefulness of traditional scientific research findings. Armed with the findings from this study, how is the nurse to tell whether patient P wants a psychosocial relationship based on primary nursing as described by Vaughan, or whether he would prefer a traditional relationship based on professional detachment of the sort advocated by Bradshaw?

And this, of course, is the point. Bradshaw might or might not be right that on a macro level, patients wish for a return to traditional, biomedically based nursing, but such an assertion can never be, as she claims, self-evident, and neither is it true for all patients in all situations. The only thing we can be certain of is that we can be certain of nothing. Patients are people and people are unique individuals. We can generalise neither from the experience of single patients such as Alice Thomas Ellis, nor from our own experiences, nor, as we have seen, from empirical studies such as that conducted by Webb and Hope.

Ironically, then, the only way that we can know whether patient P would rather be nursed holistically by a nurse-practitioner or traditionally by a nurse-technician is to ask him. And the only way that we can ask him in such a way as to be sure of an accurate and realistic answer is to engage him in a therapeutic relationship in which he feels free to respond honestly, unconstrained by the blocks to communication erected by the professionally detached nurse-technician.

So whereas Bradshaw attempted to distinguish between the physical care given by the traditional nurse and the psychosocial care of 'new nursing', arguing that they were to a large extent mutually exclusive, this book maintains that the two are inseparable, indeed that the former is dependent on the latter. If we are to respond to the unique and individual physical and biomedical needs of each patient, we must first ascertain what those needs are, and this entails getting to know our patients as individuals in what Bradshaw disparagingly referred to as 'authentic, empathic relationships of involvement'. I would certainly not wish to undermine the value of skilled, biomedical nursing and technical excellence, but it is not, as Bradshaw argued, the foundation of nursing. The foundation of nursing, if it has one, is surely the facilitative, human relationship between patient and nurse which makes skilled biomedical nursing and technical excellence possible.

New paradigm nursing as normal science

But in the face of such wide ranging resistance from the nursing establishment, how can the new paradigm ever hope to become a reality? The answer is that we have to work for change from within the existing system simply because it is the only system there is. We are constrained by having to practice in real-life clinical areas where the emphasis is often on quantity rather than quality of care; by having to apply for research funding to bodies which lay down rigid guidelines about what counts as research; by having to write curricula which impose tight professional constraints on syllabus material and assessment criteria; and by having to submit our work to journals which enforce a narrow view of academic worth and credibility.

Changes to the system will only come about from within, and a shift in the power base of the profession such as that advocated in this book will only be realised through the empowerment of practitioners with the skills, time and confidence actually to generate theory, to carry out research, to become more involved in their education, and to communicate what they are doing to others. Those of us already working in the fields of research and education must be prepared to share the power and status which our privileged positions bring with them.

If the new paradigm is to offer a serious challenge to the old, then practice, research and education initiatives need to be combined and integrated, and more importantly, demonstrated to be effective; and that requires practitioners, researchers and academics working together in equal partnership, each recognising not only their own particular skills and expertise, but those of their colleagues. Part 2 of this book offers examples from just such an initiative currently being developed in Portsmouth.

It is impossible to pinpoint where the Portsmouth initiative started. Like many innovations, it was being developed by a number of people simultaneously and in isolation from each other, with only a gradual awareness that several practitioners, researchers and lecturers were all thinking and practising along the same lines, albeit using different language to describe what they were doing. However, the eventual coming together was a creative 'AHA' experience for all concerned, exemplified in the following extract from a letter by a senior nurse specialist to a lecturer-researcher:

> For years, I thought it was me that had the problem—as so often it appeared that nursing was trying to find some solution to an insoluble problem—that patients AND nurses are human, and therefore will be different. All of a sudden, reading your words, I realised that it wasn't me that had the problem—it was nursing!

The papers in Part 2 of this book represent a selection of what has been a fruitful and mutually supportive collaboration on practice, research and educational projects, and which, we hope, form the foundations of a new paradigm in which our roles become delightfully blurred and interrelated in a concerted effort to exert a direct and beneficial influence on nursing practice and to abolish the theory-practice gap which has proved so detrimental to patient care.

References

Altrichter, H., Posch, P. and Somekh, B. (1993) *Teachers Investigate their Work*. London: Routledge.

Bateson, G. (1979) *Mind and Nature*. London: Fontana.

Bradshaw, A. (1995) What are nurses doing to patients? A review of theories of nursing past and present. *Journal of Clinical Nursing*, 4, 81–92.

Chinn, P.L. and Jacobs, M.K. (1987) *Theory and Nursing: A Systematic Approach*, 2nd edn. St Louis: Mosby.

Chinn, P.L. and Kramer, M.K. (1991) *Theory and Nursing: A Systematic Approach*, 3rd edn. St Louis: Mosby.

Darbyshire, P. (1994) Skilled expert practice: is it all in the mind? A response to English's critique of Benner's novice to expert model. *Journal of Advanced Nursing*, 19, 755–761.

Department of Health (1993) *Report of the Taskforce on the Strategy for Research in Nursing, Midwifery and Health Visiting*. London: HMSO.

Fawcett, J. (1984) *Analysis and Evaluation of Conceptual Models of Nursing*. Philadelphia: Davis.

Hollis, M. (1994) *The Philosophy of Social Science*. Cambridge: Cambridge University Press.

Hume, D. (1875) *Enquiry Concerning Human Understanding*. London: Longman.

Kuhn, T.S. (1962) *The Structure of Scientific Revolutions*. Chicago: University of Chicago Press.

Manley, K. (1991) Knowledge for nursing practice. In: *Nursing: A Knowledge Base for Practice* (A. Perry and M. Jolley, eds) London: Edward Arnold.

Meleis, A. (1985) *Theoretical Nursing: Development and Progress*. Philadelphia: Lippincott.

Pearson, A. (1988) *Primary Nursing*. London: Croom Helm.

Phillips, D.L. (1973) *Abandoning Method*. San Francisco: Jossey-Bass.

Powers, B.A. and Knapp, T.R. (1990) *A Dictionary of Nursing Theory and Research*. London: Sage.

Robinson, J. (1993) Problems with paradigms in a caring profession. In: *Nursing: Art and Science* (A. Kitson, ed.) London: Chapman and Hall.

Sayer, A. (1992) *Method in Social Science*. London: Routledge.

Vaughan, B. (1995) Celebrating 25 years of primary nursing. *Journal of Clinical Nursing*, 4, 69–70.

Walker, L.O. and Avant, K.C. (1988) *Strategies for Theory Construction in Nursing*, 2nd edn. Norwalk: Appleton and Lange.

Webb, C. and Hope, K. (1995) What kind of nurses do patients want? *Journal of Clinical Nursing*, 4, 101–108.

Williams, B.A.O. (1985) *Ethics and the Limits of Philosophy*. London: Fontana.

Ziman, J. (1978) *Reliable Knowledge*. Cambridge: Cambridge University Press.

Part 2

New paradigm nursing in action

5

Developing new roles in practice and education

Man is... nothing else but the sum of his actions, nothing else but what his life is

Jean-Paul Sartre

The shortest answer is doing

English proverb

Introduction

In the previous chapter, I discussed some of the difficulties in attempting to instigate a new paradigm for nursing within the constraints of the old. The difficulties in operating from an epistemological base and value system outside of the established norm is something which I have personally encountered in my work in education and research, but nowhere are the problems more keenly felt than in nursing practice, where nurses typically do not have the freedom or autonomy of their education colleagues to try out unorthodox ideas and new ways of working. It is unlikely, then, that the nurse–practitioner role, as I have described it, exists in its entirety anywhere at all at the present time.

This chapter examines two attempts to overcome what must at times seem like overwhelming obstacles in order to implement two very different aspects of the nurse–practitioner role. In the first, Sue Cradock reviews the developments in her role of Diabetes Nurse Specialist over the past 10 years, and describes a project to bring together clinical specialists from a variety of different areas of nursing in order to explore new ways of working. She outlines a model developed by this 'Advanced

Practice in Nursing' group which focuses on the process of nursing rather than on the content as a way of bringing together practitioners with diverse aims and needs, and demonstrates how she has applied it to the development of her own role.

In the second paper in this chapter, Moyra Skinner looks at a very different aspect of the advanced practitioner's role, the development of intuition and hypothesising as elements of nursing practice. Hypothesising was examined in Chapter 1 of this book, where it was advocated as a form of problem solving and as a component in the process of hypothetico-abductivism. Moyra's development and practical application of this approach in her own practice is a useful conformation for me that nurses can and do work in the way in which I have described. The same is true of intuition, which Moyra refers to as working from instinct, and which she describes as a normal part of advanced practice.

The third paper examines my own attempts at developing a new role for nurse educators in response to the changing economic and management structure of the health service. Once again, it recognises the huge difficulties in trying to establish a new paradigm from within the existing dominant one, and it also acknowledges the fact that within the new paradigm as proposed in this book, my own role would probably cease to exist in any recognisable form.

The final paper in this chapter describes a Level 4 research methodology, which I have referred to as grounded practice, for developing a new nursing role in response to the needs of existing service providers. In this paper, I have taken care to decontextualise the methodology. I have stripped away all references to the setting in which the role was developed, and I have deliberately not reported on the results of the study. The reason for this is that, as seen in earlier chapters, Level 3 and 4 research is not generalisable beyond the setting in which it was conducted, and the findings will not necessarily apply to other situations.

As with all Level 4 research, the primary aim of this study was to change practice, to develop a new role rather than to generate findings. What *is* generalisable, however, is the methodology, and so rather than attempting to apply the findings of this study to other settings, I would encourage colleagues to employ this methodology to generate their own findings and bring about change which is unique to their own particular setting.

The expert nurse: clinical specialist or advanced practitioner?

Sue Cradock

Background

I have been working in the role of Diabetes Nurse Specialist (DNS) for over 10 years, and whilst my title has not changed, the work that I do and the way that I do it certainly has. Prior to becoming a DNS, I had already explored the need for such a role by examining the literature, the local needs of people with diabetes, and similar developments within diabetes nursing in other areas. Although my enquiry focused mainly on the field of diabetes, I have always been interested in the development of clinical nursing beyond the traditional (as it was then) ward sister role, and therefore I also explored the role of the Clinical Nurse Specialist (CNS). In particular, I directed my attention to the work done in this field by George Castledine, who identified a number of key aspects of the CNS role. I also used the *Specialties in Nursing* report from the RCN (Royal College of Nursing, 1988) and the *Role of the Clinical Nurse Specialist* report from the ANA (American Nurses Association, 1986) to help me find the right focus for this new role.

As diabetes is centred largely within the field of medicine, there was a temptation to use the medical model to develop my role of DNS. Indeed, this is not altogether inappropriate, as there is some evidence that well-trained nurses perform routine diabetic complication screening more effectively than doctors, and also that nurses might be better placed to provide health education advice than their medical colleagues. Given the changing focus of the medical profession, there is clearly a need to develop the role of the nurse–practitioner in diabetes care to undertake these tasks, and this need is already being met by suitably trained practice nurses.

However, I chose not to develop my role along medical model lines. Initially, my work consisted primarily of developing expertise in working with people with diabetes, mainly helping them to learn the skills of diabetes self-care and to use those skills to improve both their health and their quality of life. Whilst the main thrust of my work has not changed, the way in which I work and the skills I employ undoubtedly has. At first, my practice was informed mainly by educational theory, but I now include counselling skills, psychology, empowerment models, medical skills and systems analysis, as well as providing people with information about the health care system of which they are part.

Alongside the patient-centred aspect of my work, I have also developed the role towards influencing the care provided by other health professionals to people with diabetes. Initially this was achieved through the use of training days and courses, but it quickly developed into the influencing of policies at local, district, regional and national level.

Thus, although the screening for diabetic complications and provision of health education advice is part of my work, it is by no means a major part. My problem was that of establishing the value and worth of my psychosocial, patient-centred role within a predominantly medical model of care. How could I therefore identify what I do in order that it could be valued alongside the easily identifiable medical practice skills? How could I help prevent the role of the senior nurse being seen as one of performing medical screening tests (which could be carried out by a technician) and the employment of lower grade, less experienced staff to provide the health education, promotion, provision and expertise that I am currently providing. Most importantly, how could I start to verbalise what I do by focusing on the important, relevant, effective aspects of my work?

One forum for exploring and developing my role was through a local specialist nurse group, initially set up with the aim of providing peer support for role development of these senior nursing posts. In the early years, the group was successful in fulfilling this aim, but as the posts matured and the post holders became confident in their direction and development, as well as clinically expert, the group started to become dysfunctional since there was no longer a need for the same type of support. At the same time that the group was questioning its function, there came the threat that these CNS posts were an expensive commodity that might not be really necessary.

In the midst of these internal difficulties, the UKCC intro-duced the *Post Registration Education and Practice* (PREP) report, which suggested a distinction between the roles of the Clinical Nurse Specialist (CNS) and the Advanced Nurse Practitioner (ANP). This triggered a local debate as to whether our present roles were as clinical specialists, a role which appeared to be different from that suggested by Castledine in the early 1980s, or advanced practitioners; and if they were the latter, should we be thinking of a name change? Unfortunately, the UKCC gave little guidance on what constituted the ANP role beyond the broad definition of:

> adjusting the boundaries for the development of future practice, pioneering and developing new roles responsive to changing needs and with advancing clinical practice, research and education in order to enrich professional practice as a whole. (UKCC, 1990)

A framework for expertise

All these questions and issues led to the setting up of a local 'Advanced Practice in Nursing' group, whose initial aim was to attempt to find a way of describing the role of what the UKCC referred to as advanced practitioners. Because the group was comprised of practitioners from a wide range of specialties, there were enormous problems over reaching a consensus on what exactly were the defining characteristics of advanced practice. It seemed that whatever criteria were put forward, there was always someone who did not see them as part of their role.

The group eventually resolved the problem by focusing on process rather than on content; that it is not what we do that makes us advanced practitioners, but how we do it. This approach had an amazing effect on the group; suddenly we were speaking the same language, and whilst our roles involved differ-ent content, structures and outcomes, the ways in which we worked were very similar. In particular, as advanced practition-ers we found that we were all concerned with making sense of our practice through reflection and with basing our clinical decisions to some extent on a body of personal knowledge and experience.

Having found some common ground, we quickly developed a number of 'key process criteria' in order to define and describe our roles:

1. *Clinical autonomy* — making clinical decisions based on our own clinical expertise. This involves the validation of our own expertise by exploring what it is and where it comes from, and the examination of issues such as reflection-on-action, intuition and clinical judgement in relation to expert practice.
2. *Developing clinical practice* — exploring and enhancing our own knowledge, skills and attitudes, and those of other nurses and professional colleagues. This involves the generation, acquisition and dissemination of knowledge and research findings, and the integration of formal and informal theory.
3. *Extending clinical boundaries* — moving the boundaries within the defined area of nursing of the individual practitioner. In some cases this will involve extending the scope of what nurses do, both medically and psychosocially, and in other cases it might mean rejecting existing roles as inappropriate.
4. *Defining a clinical focus* — a specialty within a specialty. This is related to the above criterion and involves developing an eclectic role within what might be a narrow specialty. As nursing grows ever more technical and complex, expertise can increasingly only be achieved at the expense of breadth of knowledge and skill.
5. *Influencing local and national policies and politics* — having an impact which extends beyond our clinical areas.

It can be seen that this framework is essentially a process model which individuals can apply to their specialist area, unlike other definitions of advanced and specialist practice which specify content such as research, management and teaching knowledge and skills. It therefore attempts to combine the models of the CNS and the ANP by expanding and developing the role of the nurse within the context of her own specialty. As CNSs, each of the group members has a specialist body of knowledge, theory and skills in their own chosen clinical field, but they also have a shared approach to generating and applying knowledge, theory and skills which defines them as advanced practitioners as well as specialists. In many ways, the above criteria outline a role similar to that defined by Benner as an expert, that is, a nurse who has developed a specialist body of skills and knowledge through prolonged experience in a particular clinical setting, but who also possesses an intuitive 'know-how' that comes from sustained and methodical reflection on her own practice.

Applying the framework

The diabetes specialist nursing team have already started work using this model, and I will now demonstrate some of the ways in which the above framework can be employed to structure and describe the work of the expert nurse in this one particular area of care, although the framework can, of course, be applied to any nursing specialty.

Clinical autonomy

Clinical autonomy in diabetes nursing involves not only making decisions about appropriate care, but also about the most appropriate carer. To take an example, a patient referred by a medical practitioner to the CNS to be taught blood glucose monitoring was not very keen to learn this skill. On assessment by the CNS, the duration of the diabetes, the complication status and the lack of 'osmotic' symptoms suggested that the patient was not at major risk of deterioration in health, and the CNS therefore agreed with the patient that the skill of blood glucose monitoring was not appropriate. However, there was evidence of a slightly raised blood glucose level which could be improved by increasing the quality of carbohydrate in the patient's diet, and therefore a referral was made to the specialist dietician. It is recognised that this kind of intervention goes beyond the normal remit of the nurse, and required a change in local policy (see the section on influencing local and national policies and politics below).

Developing clinical practice

In the field of diabetes nursing, this involves identifying the potential advanced practice skills in other nurses and acting in a professional mentoring role to support those individuals' development, often outside of the formal organisational structure; as well as offering mentorship to other professional colleagues such as doctors, dieticians and podiatrists. It also involves providing information, advice and structured education sessions to colleagues regarding appropriate diabetes care.

In order to develop our own knowledge base for clinical practice, it is necessary to effectively combine formal and informal knowledge and theory. For example, a recent major research study conclusively demonstrated that good blood glucose control reduces the risk of microvascular complications over a 10 year period. The challenge for nurse–practitioners is now to interpret and apply those findings to our own individual practice, where it is well accepted that only a proportion of people with diabetes can achieve good control.

We also have to work with research data that gives us average information regarding insulin actions and regimens, since all insulin action graphs are descriptions of the mean dose response curve. But most diabetes clinicians will know from experience that individual variation is great, and we must therefore call on our tacit, personal knowledge of our individual patients when they fall outside of the expected norms provided by formal research studies. Research-based clinical practice is therefore an integration of global, generalisable, 'average' research data with personal, unique, specific knowledge of individual patients.

Extending clinical boundaries

I stated earlier that I do not see the role of the DSN as taking over unwanted tasks from the medical team, for example, routine complications screening. Rather, the DSN should be concerned with extending herself as a nurse, and there are a number of ways that our team has attempted to do this.

Firstly, all patients being referred to the consultant are initially seen by a DSN, who not only assesses current and future care and clinical needs, but also attempts to explain and clarify the system of care so that the patient can make the best use of his consultation. In this way, any immediate changes in care can be initiated prior to the medical consultation, including referral to a dietician or retinal screening service, instigation of blood glucose monitoring, the alteration or commencement of medication, for example, insulin or oral hypoglycaemic agents, as well as education and counselling.

While it could be argued that all of the above, especially the prescription of medication, are medical roles, I would argue that they fall very much within the nurse's domain, being concerned with the day-to-day care and well-being of the patient. Furthermore, the nursing assessment is not supplementary to the appointment with the consultant, but is an integral part of the overall care package. The nurse is not taking on a role discarded by the medical team, but is employing her unique clinical skills in areas which she can perform *better* than her medical colleagues.

Secondly, the DSN draws on her counselling and educational skills as well as her expert knowledge of medical interventions in assisting the patient to understand the rationale for certain treatment or management strategies. In this way, many patients who might have refused treatment can be helped to make an informed choice. It should be emphasised that the nurse is not an apologist for the medical and management staff, but an autonomous practitioner who is utilising her unique relationships with her patients to ensure that they receive the best possible treatment.

Defining a clinical focus

The DSN team has developed a clearly defined role within the field of diabetes care without setting up immovable boundaries, and within the team, each member has identified a specific area of care on which to focus their interest and research, including professional education, acute in-patient care, primary health-care support, pregnancy and foot ulcer management. This identification of specialties within the parent specialty encourages the development of advanced practice without detracting from the continuity of care for the patient, since each DSN is able to provide her patients with the appropriate expert care by calling upon the expertise of her colleagues in a consultancy fashion.

Influencing local and national policies and politics

Challenges to national policies often start at a local level, and can take several forms. First and most straightforwardly, by being aware of local population needs, political influences and health-care changes, we are formulating plans to develop present services more appropriately to meet local needs.

Secondly, we are challenging national nursing opinion and practice by initiating local agreements. For example, dieticians traditionally only accept referrals from a registered medical practitioner, but this has caused local delays in patients receiving appropriate dietary advice. We have therefore negotiated an agreement that allows the DSN to refer patients to dieticians directly, and this has proved so successful that it has recently been expanded to include practice nurses in community settings. Thus, while there has been no change nationally in the professional stance of dieticians, the direct access by nurses to dieticians has been achieved by initiating locally agreed team protocols.

And thirdly, general, non-diabetes-specific policies have been challenged as inappropriate to the care of patients with diabetes, for example in the use of certain types of syringes and in the local system of assessing and recording clinical activity.

Conclusion

This is only the beginning of the development of a process model for expert practice. The framework described earlier was built up from the experiences of the 'Advanced Practice in Nursing' group, and our attempt to apply it to the field of diabetes nursing is yet to be fully validated by exposure to health service managers, to nurse theorists, and, of course, to practising nurses, over a protracted period of time.

Although a recommendation of PREP, not all the specialist nurses and advanced practitioners in the group have a degree or are even in the process of studying for one, and not all would necessarily see their advanced or specialist role in the way described in the PREP report. However, from discussions about using the above model, the attraction of describing their work in terms of process is clearly evident, not least because it enables communication across the most diverse of specialties. The next stage in the implementation, both in diabetes nursing and more generally, is therefore to develop skills in reflective practice, process analysis of nursing activities and professional supervision, with the eventual goal of being able to define, evaluate and enhance advanced nursing practice.

References

American Nurses Association (1986) *The Role of the Clinical Nurse Specialist*. Missouri: American Nurses Association.

Royal College of Nursing (1988) *Specialties in Nursing. Working Party report*. London: RCN.

UKCC (1990) *Report of the Post-Graduate Practice Project*. London: UKCC.

The role of hypothesising and intuition in advanced practice

Moyra Skinner and Gary Rolfe

Introduction

This paper takes the form of two excerpts from an interview I conducted with Moyra Skinner, a trained psychiatric nurse and family therapist. In the first, Moyra describes the methods common in family therapy work of hypothesising and live supervision, and in the second, she explores her experiences of what she calls working from instinct. Both excerpts are followed by commentaries in which I attempt to locate Moyra's insights and experiences within the framework and terminology of this book.

Excerpt 1: hypothesising and live supervision

Can you tell me a bit about the method of hypothesising in family therapy work?

For me, it's a very good way of learning to work from the basis of a hypothesis and then testing it out, modifying it or rejecting it totally, and that can give some very important and powerful structure to your work, not only with families but with individual clients as well. And for me, it's more about using whatever information you have, either from the referral or other knowledge of the person. That initial meeting gives you some more human feedback in terms of their behaviour with each other, what the different agendas are for each of them, and their perceptions; there are always different perceptions for each of them of what's going on, and what each of them is doing with that perception.

The hypothesis can either be on a fairly superficial level about their ability or not to negotiate, their ability or not to acknowledge their own part in the difficulty, or it can be on a much more profound level which is more about the heavier dynamics of their current families and previous relationships or family of origin, which may be affecting what's happening now; in other words, the baggage they carry.

You said that the hypothesis is formed from your assessment of the person, from how much you know about them. To what extent do you use your more formal knowledge of psychiatry?

A great deal, in terms of people's defences and coping strategies. As you get more skilled it becomes easier to identify what are people's main ones: is it about denial; are they rationalising; are they projecting? So yes, my knowledge of psychiatry and quite intensive individual work is hugely valuable because that enables a much deeper level of perception. And thinking about the next part of the hypothesis, I can obviously check that out with colleagues from other disciplines and other perceptions, which again is very useful.

So it's a combination of textbook knowledge and personal knowledge of that person?

Yes.

Can you just talk through the process of hypothesising?

We rarely get a very in-depth referral, it tends to be fairly minimal information, but I don't find that too much of a disadvantage, in fact I find it quite positive, because my belief is that you have to work with what the couple or family brings; it's no good working with your agenda, it has to be theirs. People are always there by choice, they are adults, and just by being there they are making a statement that they want to do something different; what they have done to date has stopped working. In terms of the information, it's about asking them what is happening for them now, how they perceive what's happening now, and what's problematic about it. And then, on that information, it's possible, particularly with live supervision, to come up with a working hypothesis, which you then go back and in some measure feed back to the clients. I said 'in some measure' not to patronise them by implying they don't know what they're talking about, but from the point of view of opening things up for them; I think if you swamp people with information you tend to scare them away, but it's about reflecting some of what we see, about how they are, their behaviour, and reflecting back what we believe that means.

Could you give an example?

We worked with a couple from a different culture. He has a professional qualification and runs his own business, and his wife was the person with the original 'identified problem', that is, depression. Despite a period of individual work for her, little changed and we were asked to see them.

One of the most obvious differences we noticed when we first met with them was their very different ways of dealing with problems and with each other. He was very concrete, factual and logical, very much involved in the process, while she was totally wrapped up in the content, emotion and thoughts. Because they were both so entrenched in their positions, increasingly so as they became more threatened, the communication gap became even wider and the only way they were able to bridge it was loudly with rows and arguments.

We fed this back to them. Our hypothesis was that for whatever reason they had stopped communicating effectively; it was clear that they had at some point, but for some reason they had stopped. We didn't know why, so we just fed back to them that for some reason their communication had got stuck and had floundered. We gave them a small task about spending some time together and just talking, but without any negative feedback, which they did. We thought a lot about why they had got so stuck and why she had remained fairly chronically depressed. We hypothesised that it might have something to do with the different ways they were dealing with their cultural expectations in a different country: he was very much wanting to be very 'English', but clearly the family culture was very important to her and her role within it. It seemed she had more of a dilemma about where her responsibilities and loyalties were; he was much more western about that.

The next time we saw them, that was one of the things we fed back to them, and that unstoppered things in that they were then able to tell us about lots of difficulties, almost all around the family, but also about them. They are very different. She had become very caught up in some destructive relationships within their large extended family and had responded on a strong emotional level. Her inability to step out of the 'content' and use a process to untangle the situation led eventually to much distress between them. The distress and entrenchment in their individual positions and perceptions has lasted for several years; they seemed to be looking at each other from opposite shores.

So that expanded our hypothesis a bit more, which was that somehow his feelings about the situation had remained unresolved and she carried them. We fed that back to them and said that he needed to learn from her about getting in touch with his emotions, but perhaps one of the things he could help her to learn was to compartmentalise things a bit, that is, create some different boundaries that made things more manageable for her. So it was a lot about them communicating about abilities and skills that they both had and needed to share.

Do you always feed back the hypothesis, or do you sometimes just make inferences or interpretations from them and work with those?

It would very much depend on the people.

The kind of process you are describing seems to be this: you have a hypothesis, you somehow put it into action, either by feeding it back or by suggesting a task, and then you assess the impact of that, and either change your hypothesis or develop it more, and it's a process.

Oh yes, very much so.

But one of the ways of testing out a hypothesis is simply to share it with them and see what they think.

And depending on people's ability to use abstract ideas or not; some people need to work in abstract ways, so you need to adapt how you feed that back. Sometimes you can be very straightforward, and sometimes it's necessary to make the messages smaller and more spread out.

You mentioned live supervision just now. Can you say a bit more about it?

Live supervision is the process where one or more therapists is in the room with the clients and one or more is outside the room observing through a one-way screen or video camera, so they are able to see things from a different perspective. The person in the room picks up the emotion, and the very close things that you get from people, whereas the person who is observing is able to see a much broader picture. If the observer believes you are being diverted, they can call you out and say 'we think this is happening. Whatever it was you touched on is uncomfortable and you need to go back to it'. Or 'what we see happening is...' and they will describe somebody's changing body posture or demeanour at some particular point which, if you happen to be addressing another member of the family, you could well miss, because you have to keep people engaged. So it's different levels of information, and when you meet together towards the end of the session to discuss what's going on, you have all of that. It's like a three-dimensional picture rather than something flat, and rather than going away and thinking about it and saving it for cold supervision as perhaps one does with individual work, it is live, you're there while it's happening, so you can respond very quickly.

Do the people behind the screen take part in the process of hypothesising?

Yes

So they might call you out and suggest a hypothesis?

Yes. The hypothesis generally comes about through discussion, with all of you giving information, ideas and perceptions.

So hypotheses are normally formulated outside of the situation, rather than, say, the primary worker coming up with a hypothesis.

Yes, I think it's a mixture. Sometimes there is a situation where the primary therapist will come out and say 'I don't know what's going on in there'. It may well be that you are so swamped by the high expressed emotion in the room that all you can manage to deal with is that, which is why it's so valuable to have somebody outside. They can say 'what was happening was...', and they can actually describe the process of the session, which in conjunction with your experience in there, can give you a very valid picture. As with the couple described earlier, sometimes content and process lose touch with each other.

Commentary

Although Moyra is describing the technique of hypothesising from the perspective of family therapy work, it is essentially an approach to problem solving and can therefore be applied to any nursing intervention where there is a clinical problem to be resolved. Moyra employs a combination of formal theory, for example the theory of psychological defence mechanisms, and informal theory derived from personal knowledge about the individual client. However, she makes it clear that of the two, the most important source of information is what the clients bring with them rather than the therapist's own agenda. The process being described is therefore very similar to the method of abduction described in Chapter 1: the therapist works primarily from what she knows of the individual client, but employs formal theory in formulating the most appropriate hypothesis.

The example given by Moyra clearly illustrates the way in which hypotheses are tested out in practice and refined as a result. Moyra's initial hypothesis of a communication breakdown was very general, and offered no attempt at an explanation. It was fed back to the clients without analysis or interpretation, and was tested out clinically by giving the couple the simple task of spending time together talking. This intervention modified the clinical situation, leading to a new assessment and a refined hypothesis that the couple were dealing with problems in different and incompatible ways.

The new hypothesis was tested by feeding it back to the clients, and its accuracy was confirmed by its clinical effect of 'unstoppering' the communication block. The clinical situation was therefore modified further since the couple were now communicating, and as a result of this enhanced dialogue, Moyra and her team were able to refine the hypothesis further: that the husband had not resolved his feelings about his wife's involvement in the family chaos. This new hypothesis was then fed back, more tasks were set, and so on in a continuing cycle.

In this example, hypotheses were tested and practice modified either simply by sharing the hypothesis with the clients, or by actively changing the clinical situation by setting a task. These two methods are particularly suited to family therapy work, and nurses working in other clinical settings would have to find their own ways of testing hypotheses, probably by making some sort of clinical intervention.

Finally, live supervision was briefly discussed. This is another specific family therapy technique, but one which would be very difficult to apply to other areas of nursing practice. However, its scope as a method of training nurses in reflection-in-action is enormous. Nurses could practise on-the-spot experimenting in role-play situations, with observers sitting behind a screen and calling out the nurse to suggest hypotheses and interventions, which could then be tried out immediately in practice.

Excerpt 2: working from instinct

So what about this idea of working from instinct?

I called it instinct for a long time and got hassle from various supervisors, who kept on saying 'that's not what it is, you actually know that something's the case, or have decided that such and such is the case, based on some knowledge that you have somewhere. The way to access that is to work it back in supervision: how did you know that, how did you get to that understanding?'. I've been doing that more and more, and have decided that they are right, and it's not just a leap of faith because that would be very dangerous and unprofessional. The sense of things that I have is very powerful, but because of lots of experience in a variety of areas, both personal and professional, I have learnt to trust them, but then I have to make sense of them.

Why do you have to make sense of them? Do you make sense of them afterwards?

Increasingly I am able to make sense of them at the time. That process of tracking back has become more immediate for me, I don't have to search for it quite so much. I think it was quite difficult for a long time trying to identify the process, going backwards. But as I hung in there and really worked hard at doing that, I am able to go through the process quite quickly.

What are these instincts based on?

They are based on past experiences and the information that we store with each experience.

Are they based on specific past experiences?

Many of them, or on collections of experiences.

But you can actually recall the experiences they are based on?

Yes, some of them.

You said that you no longer work from these instincts without analysing them, and that nowadays...

I think the analysis nowadays is happening as I'm saying it, or even just before.

So would you see that as a progression in the way you work?

Oh, absolutely, I can remember very early on when I was practising, being pretty clear in my head that this was the right way to respond, and sometimes in sessions thinking 'where did that come from?', being quite surprised at what I came out with.

And did you then go back afterwards and figure out where it came from?

Yes, I would go back, particularly in supervision, and question it, and I think I struggled with that for a while. But then with supervision, I got some direction as to what it was about, and how I could more consciously access it.

I guess that's what Schön calls reflection-on-action: that you do it and go away afterwards and figure out why you do it, and figure out where the information came from.

Sure, and that is a building-up of my personal store of knowledge and information.

But now you work differently.

Yes, I think that there is still that reflection-on-action, but it's much more immediate, it's more reflection-in-action.

Benner gives examples of nurses working from intuition, and they are almost doing it on automatic, they seem very detached from the situation. Is it the same for you?

No, I honestly don't think that necessarily makes you very good at what you do. You have to have some involvement because we are all human beings, and we all have the potential for the same feelings.

What about your state of awareness? Are you detached from it and working on auto-pilot?

Yes, I suppose to an extent, in that I am able to... I am certainly in a state of heightened awareness. It's a bit like sharpening the focus in those situations. Particularly in very stressful, very critical situations, it's just like sharpening the focus and I become aware of everything. Their changing body language, their language, all sorts of things.

So it's very much focused in the here and now?

Yes, because those situations are very critical, but I am also thinking about computing the subtle changes I am seeing in front of me, making some assessment about what that means and some decision about how to respond, as it's happening, very quickly.

Commentary

What Moyra describes as instinct is clearly very similar to Benner's account of intuition, that is, a manifestation of expertise, and the fact that it was recognised as such by her supervisors suggests that it is by no means uncommon amongst nurses. It is interesting that she felt the need to work backwards in supervision to discover where this instinct came from, presumably to validate her actions and to build up her 'personal store of knowledge and information', what Benner referred to as a repertoire of paradigm cases.

More interesting, however, is Moyra's statement that she no longer has to do this because she can now make sense of it at the time. She has progressed from reflection-on-action to reflection-in-action. Her problem solving has become a conscious process very similar to that described in Chapter 3 as advanced practice, in which the nurse is concentrating on every action, every clinical decision rather than operating on auto-pilot. Moyra describes this as sharpening the focus to the point where she is aware of everything that is happening, and she ends with a perfect description of reflection-in-action as 'thinking about computing the subtle changes I am seeing in front of me, making some assessment about what that means and some decision about how to respond, as it's happening, very quickly'.

A new role for the nurse educator

Gary Rolfe

The changing face of nurse education

The move towards a technocratic model has resulted in many radical changes in nurse education, including the Project 2000 curriculum, the integration of colleges of nursing into higher education, and the new purchaser–provider relationship between the trusts as purchasers of education and schools as providers. The introduction of Project 2000 and the resulting demand for the teaching of a wider knowledge base has initiated a move away from the generic course tutor role towards that of a subject specialist, and the move into higher education has reinforced this shift with a change in title from tutor to lecturer.

This latter change in particular is having a profound effect on the relationship between educators and practitioners. No longer are they part of the same professional group; they are separate professions with separate agendas, and this has important implications for how they perceive and relate to one another. In addition, the purchaser–provider arrangement makes educators accountable to their colleagues in practice as never before.

These changes have resulted in competing demands on the providers of nurse education. On the one hand, a great deal of teaching is now driven by the contracts with the trusts, leading in many cases to increased student contact hours and an emphasis on clinically based teaching. On the other hand, however, the universities and colleges into which schools of nursing are moving consider the pursuit of scholarly activities such as publishing, speaking at conferences and generating income from research to be a necessary part of the role of the lecturer.

Responding to the changes

A truly post-technocratic model of education would necessarily blur the distinctions between practitioner and lecturer, thereby solving many of our current problems, but unfortunately we are forced to work within the existing technocratic model, and as educators we must respond to the challenges it throws up as best we can. The dilemma that these dual demands from trust and university are imposing on lecturers in schools of nursing and health studies is forcing us to look at our role as never before, and to ask ourselves the question: *What does it mean to be a lecturer within the higher education system in a discipline that is primarily practice based?*

This is a personal response to that question: as a former nurse tutor, and since 1992, a lecturer in healthcare research, I wish to argue that my role is *not* the same as that of a lecturer in a theory based discipline, but neither is it the same as that of the traditional nurse tutor. Rather, it is a new and different role that is up to us as a profession to define. Somehow, we must satisfy the needs of the trusts we are contracted to, meet our commitments as traditional university lecturers, and also provide education that is relevant to the needs of the post-technocratic nurse–practitioner. I believe that there are many possible solutions to this dilemma, and that it is important that we explore a broad range of different roles.

There is a powerful and convincing lobby within nurse education for the lecturer to maintain her clinical involvement, and there are two commonly held views as to why this is important. On the one hand, there is the argument for clinical *credibility*, that in order to teach *nurses*, lecturers must present as credible nurses themselves. On the other hand, there is the argument for clinical *expertise*, that in order to teach *nursing*, lecturers must themselves be experts in practice.

These are both compelling arguments, and I would particularly concur with the latter, that to teach nursing skills at anything above a basic level, lecturers must possess an expertise in those skills based on a body of personal knowledge and theory generated from reflection on clinical experience. Whereas clinical credibility can be maintained by spending as little as half-a-day per week in a clinical practice setting, expertise clearly requires a more intensive involvement, and the lecturer–practitioner role is perhaps the most appropriate model for the teacher of advanced clinical skills.

However, for those of us with subject specialisms such as research methods, sociology or psychology, who teach nurses rather that nursing, the lecturer–practitioner model, and even the arrangement of 1 day per week in clinical practice, is totally inappropriate. And while from the perspective of a post-technocratic model of education it might not be appropriate to teach these subjects as distinct and separate from nursing, we are all constrained to some extent by the Project 2000 curriculum and its commitment to technocratic education. We must therefore acknowledge that practising clinical nurses are the experts in nursing, that our practical expertise is as educators rather than as nurses, and that our repertoire of paradigm cases, our body of skills and know-how, is in the field of educational practice rather than of clinical practice.

I am aware that this view is unpopular with many of my colleagues who wish to maintain their professional status as nurses, and those who teach nursing rather than nurses are justified in their objections. However, as we move fully into higher education, we are confronted with a choice of whether we remain in the nursing profession or join the lecturing profession. It is a stark choice that each one of us has to make as an individual, but I believe that those of us who choose education should do so wholeheartedly.

In many ways, I relinquished my role as a nurse when I moved into education: now I have chosen, albeit reluctantly, to give up the profession of nursing. I now see myself primarily as a lecturer in higher education, but as a lecturer with particular needs and difficulties, since the majority of my teaching is to students from a practice-based discipline who must apply what I teach to clinical situations. Furthermore, although I relinquished the profession of nurse voluntarily, the PREP regulations on re-registration will mean that at least some of my colleagues might be forced down the same path against their wishes.

A new model for the lecturer of nurses

For people in my position, there is a clear need for an alternative to the traditional model of clinical links with service colleagues, which both satisfies our contractual requirements with the trusts and meets the challenges involved in developing a career as an educator rather than as a nurse. The key for me to this delicate balancing act is in satisfying the trusts that they are getting value for money, while at the same time satisfying myself that I am making a valued and worthwhile contribution to clinical practice and patient care, albeit vicariously.

From my own experience of talking with senior nurses and trust managers, it would appear that what they want from lecturers is firstly, more clinical teaching and more tutors in clinical areas, and secondly, more courses with a strong clinical skills base. Furthermore, they have made it quite clear that we are operating in a market economy, and if we do not provide the services they require, they will purchase them elsewhere. However, as this book has attempted to argue, nurses themselves are best placed to provide those services, and while the traditional clinical role of the nurse tutor is undeniably appropriate for some of my colleagues, I find it unacceptable for myself not only for the reasons stated earlier, but also because it is out of keeping with the philosophy of nursing and education outlined in this book. It makes the assumption that nursing knowledge is academically based and is handed down from teacher to pupil, whereas it is being argued here that, on the contrary, much valuable knowledge is generated *in* practice and *from* practice through the process of reflection on experience. Furthermore, if this model of nursing knowledge is accepted, then the presence of a lecturer in a clinical area imparting knowledge to students and practitioners is likely to widen rather than reduce the theory–practice gap.

In addition, my own nursing practice (and, I suspect, that of many of my colleagues) is undeniably rusty, and my personal clinical knowledge-base is rather outdated. I am no longer an expert practitioner, and would certainly not wish to be viewed as a role model. As I stated earlier, my profession is now as a lecturer, not a nurse, although I hope I have an insight into the needs and problems of nurses. I therefore wish to argue that we should be pro-active, and not merely respond to the demands of trust managers who may be unaware of what we as a profession have to offer. Our role should go beyond teaching. We should fully utilise our skills and personal knowledge as academics as well as our training as nurses to provide a useful and practical service to the trusts, whilst at the same time meeting our commitments as lecturers in higher education, and playing a full part in the academic life of the college or university which is now our employer.

What follows is my personal response to the diverse demands placed on me by my local Healthcare Trust and my University. As such, it is an attempt to develop an academic role which maintains meaningful clinical involvement outside the traditional model of clinical contact. This new role has several components: the education of students, the education of trained staff, and academic support.

The education of students

This model argues that the focus of education in the clinical setting should be clinical. It is an opportunity for students to learn both from experience through their contact with patients, and from the transmission of the personal, internalised knowledge of the practitioners. It is therefore important that the majority of the students' education in clinical areas is provided by practising nurses from those clinical areas, since the personal, tacit knowledge of the non-practising lecturer relates to education rather than to nursing.

Benner (1984) argued that expertise involves an intuition that is based on a repertoire of past paradigm cases. Experience is essential in developing such a repertoire, but equally important is reflection on that experience. The role of the lecturer in this process is in externalising and formalising the experience gained in clinical areas through the facilitation of reflective practice and critical incident analysis in the classroom. These are high level cognitive abilities, involving synthesis, analysis and evaluation, and their facilitation in students demands great educational expertise. It is therefore an appropriate role for the lecturer in her educational partnership with practitioners, requiring a unique combination of skills in the practice of education, together with an empathic understanding of the practice of nursing.

There will, of course, be objections that this model of clinically based education is too demanding of time on the practitioner, but I believe that the decision to offer a clinical setting as a training area should not be taken lightly, and that quality education is very time intensive.

Education of trained staff

The focus of this part of the role is on lifelong learning, on learning how to learn. The emphasis is therefore on the *process* of learning rather than on content, and includes working with trained staff on:

- how to access knowledge — the use of libraries and information technology;
- how to generate knowledge — reflective practice, research methods;
- how to process knowledge — critically reading academic papers, extracting relevant information;
- how to apply knowledge — putting theory into practice, hypothesising;
- how to disseminate knowledge — written and oral presentations.

The other part of the role of the lecturer in the education of trained staff is teaching how to teach. This includes the skills of teaching in clinical areas, such as facilitation, clinical supervision, reflective practice and critical incident analysis, as well as the skills of teaching in formal settings. These latter skills are important since I believe that practising nurses have a far greater role to play than at present in the teaching of clinically based courses, including many ENB courses.

Academic support

Teaching is only part of the extended role of the lecturer, and she also possesses a number of other skills and attributes of great value to her clinical colleagues:

- *Research Skills* are particularly valuable in the current market economy, where healthcare providers are having to justify their treatment approaches in terms of clinical outcomes.
- *Writing Skills* are similarly important for disseminating the work of the clinical areas and attracting publicity to examples of good practice.

- The *Ability to Access Funding* combines the skills of writing and research. The lecturer is not only able to write funding proposals in the appropriate academic language, but has access to funding opportunities, particularly research grants, from her university or institute of higher education, from charities, from the Economic and Social Research Council, from Regional funds, and from the Department of Health.
- *Academic Credibility* can be lent to good clinical work that might otherwise go unrecognised.
- *Contacts and Collaborations* are opened up beyond the immediate confines of the clinical setting, with access to a different, wider network.
- *Resources* such as audio-visual aids, information technology, libraries and classroom space can also be made available.

Conclusion

The move to a technocratic model of nurse education has resulted in a split between teachers of nursing and teachers of supporting disciplines such as sociology, psychology, law, ethics and life science. Whereas in the early days of Project 2000, the majority of this supporting material was taught by lecturers from disciplines outside nursing, much of it is now being covered by nurses themselves, and I believe that they must decide whether they wish to remain as nurses with an expertise in nursing practice and theory, or to become lecturers with an expertise in educational practice and theory. Of course, some might wish to argue that they have a theoretical expertise in nursing and a practical expertise in education, but I have argued in this book that theory and practice cannot be separated in this way, that they are two sides of the same coin of praxis.

Although nursing has been committed to higher education for some years now, we are only just beginning to appreciate the full impact of this move from a pre-technocratic to a technocratic model of education, with the competing demands of clinical practice and academia. Many of my colleagues are trying to straddle both worlds; attempting to maintain a degree of clinical expertise while at the same time meeting the need for research, publications, and general scholarly activity demanded by the academic community.

It is my belief that this route will end in disaster, that both are (more than) full-time activities, and that by attempting both we will do justice to neither. I do not believe that the model of spending 1 day per week in clinical practice can result in lecturers who are also expert nurses; at best this model can endow us with some clinical credibility in the eyes of our students, but no more than that. And anything more than 1 day per week in practice and we begin to lose our academic expertise.

I maintain that we should embrace the split between nurses and educationalists, and should make a firm commitment to one side or the other. The model proposed here outlines one way forward for educationalists who are teachers of nurses rather than of nursing, and advocates the forming of partnerships with our clinical colleagues in which both groups utilise their theoretical and practical expertise to their mutual benefit and to the benefit of their students. This entails recognising that practising nurses are best equipped to teach practical nursing skills, and that, among other things, educators are best placed to facilitate reflection on that practice and the generation of personal knowledge and informal theory. And as well as satisfying the demands of a technocratic model of education, this role is also a useful blueprint for a post-technocratic model, if or when it ever becomes accepted in nursing.

Reference

Benner, P. (1984) *From Novice to Expert*. California: Addison-Wesley.

Developing and evaluating the role of a nurse–practitioner

Gary Rolfe

Introduction

This research project was designed to develop and evaluate a new role of a nurse–practitioner inductively from first principles. The project had two aims: firstly, to create a new nursing role within an existing service, based on the needs and wants of the practitioners already working in that service; and secondly, to make an impact on the current provision of care.

The philosophy underpinning the project was that new nursing roles should be developed in response to perceived need at grassroots level rather than by managers or academics who have limited clinical experience and who might well be out of touch with the current needs of patients and practitioners. The methodology therefore has much in common with the grounded theory approach to research, the discovery of theory from data through the method of theoretical sampling (Glaser and Strauss, 1967). This method requires the researcher to start by collecting data based only on a general sociological perspective and on a general subject or problem area rather than on a preconceived theoretical framework, and to build theory from the bottom up in response to ongoing data analysis.

However, whereas Glaser and Strauss, as sociologists, were concerned with the construction of theory, this project had as its aim the development of practice, and might therefore be described as a 'grounded practice' approach to research. In keeping with this philosophy, the new post was not advertised with a job description, but with a very loose person specification calling for a graduate nurse with relevant clinical and research experience.

This philosophy of developing and expanding the role of the nurse as a result of empirical research findings is consistent with the UKCC's vision of advanced nursing practice as being 'concerned with adjusting the boundaries for the development

of future practice, pioneering and developing new roles responsive to changing needs....' (UKCC, 1994). The post was therefore
advertised with the title of Advanced Nurse Practitioner (ANP),
although this reflects the terminology adopted by the UKCC
rather than that adopted in Chapter 3 of this book, of a reflexive
practitioner working beyond Benner's level of expert.

Project philosophy

The project was conceived as a participative action research
initiative in which the role of the ANP was to be developed and
refined over a period of 18 months to meet the needs of existing
service providers, but also in response to the reflection-on-
action of the ANP herself. Thus, although essentially a Level 4
action research project, it also incorporated Level 3 reflective
methods.

It will be recalled from Chapter 2 that Usher and Bryant (1989)
stipulated four criteria for action research. It is, they claimed,
research which:

• is carried out by practitioners, or at least, that researchers are
  actually participating in the practices being researched, and
  working collaboratively with practitioners;
• improves practice through transformation of the practice
  situation;
• involves a process of reflection on, and understanding of,
  action and its outcomes, and of acting through understanding;
• is systematic in its approach, and is open to public scrutiny
  and critique.

(from Usher and Bryant, 1989)

This project met all of the above criteria by being carried out by
practitioners themselves, in this case, by the Advanced Nurse
Practitioner and a research nurse who worked in the unit where
the ANP was based; by transforming the practice situation through
the introduction of the new post of ANP as part of the research
project; by involving the ANP in reflecting on her practice and
modifying her role accordingly; and by publicly reporting on the

methodology and findings of the project through journal publications, conferences, and in-house presentations.

However, as Usher and Bryant pointed out, the action researcher-practitioner is not content merely to carry out the research study and publish the findings; this approach to research seeks to bring about change as part of the research process itself. Furthermore, the Level 4 researcher does not want to bring about just any change, but change felt to be desirable. In the words of Schön (1983) 'the practitioner has an interest in transforming the situation from what it is to something he likes better'.

Level 4 research is therefore, by its very nature, subjective, since the changes that it attempts to bring about are changes which are considered desirable by the researcher. That is not to say, however, that the researcher will approach the study with an anticipation of the findings; rather that she will have a notion of what constitutes desirable change in the situation under investigation.

In the case of this project, the researchers did not have any clear ideas or preconceptions about the role of the Advanced Nurse Practitioner that would emerge, only that they wished to bring about positive and desirable change in patient care. Arguably, this is the main advantage to Level 4 research: whereas the objective, scientific, external researcher attempts to remain neutral to the situation under examination, the Level 4 researcher brings with her an agenda to improve practice, and a body of professional knowledge and experience as to exactly what improved practice means, and this agenda shapes and directs the research.

Project design

The project was designed in three phases (Figure 5.1):

Phase 1 — assessment of needs

This first phase of the project lasted for 3 months, and was designed to ascertain the perceived needs and expectations of relevant healthcare workers with regard to the new Advanced

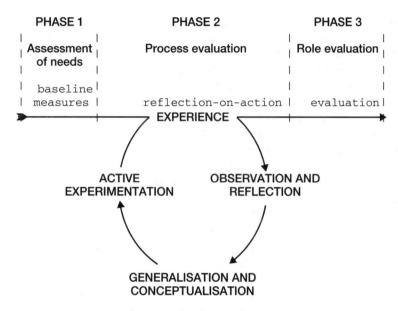

Figure 5.1 The design of the study

Nurse Practitioner role. Semi-structured group workshops were held with a wide range of professional, support, and voluntary workers (*n*=42), including hospital managers, ward-based and community nurses, occupational therapists, social workers, hospital based doctors, GPs and private sector workers and managers. The findings were content analysed and used to construct a provisional job description for the ANP, thereby ensuring that the role was responsive to the needs of the service.

Data concerning the anticipated positive effects (hopes) and negative effects (fears) of the implementation of the role of the ANP were also collected. These data were important for two reasons: firstly, the hopes and fears of the healthcare workers impinging on the role of the ANP had to be addressed and responded to if the ANP was to successfully integrate into the team; and secondly, the findings would serve as valuable baseline data when the project was evaluated in Phase 3. At the end of this first phase, the ANP came into post.

Phase 2 — process evaluation

The second phase lasted for 12 months, and was designed to evaluate and modify the role of the ANP while she was in post, in response to the changing needs of the service users. This was achieved through a process of reflection-on-action, whereby the ANP kept a reflective diary of her work, including critical incident analysis, and took part in regular in-depth interviews with the project research nurse.

By constantly monitoring her work, the ANP was able to reflect on her experiences and interventions, generalise and conceptualise from those reflections, and modify her practice accordingly in an experiential learning cycle (Kolb and Fry, 1975). In this way, a dynamic, immediately responsive role was developed, grounded in the needs and requirements of the service users and providers.

This phase of the project, during which the ANP was in post, was the most action-oriented. Thus, although the reflective interviews were recorded, the aim was not to produce transcripts for later analysis, but for the ANP to reflect on her past practice in order to formulate action plans for the future. The transcripts were merely a record of the way in which the role developed, illustrating the thoughts, feelings and frustrations of the ANP, along with her perceptions of her working relationships with other professionals.

A number of quite major modifications to the role were introduced as a result of the ANP's reflection-on-action, but it must be remembered that what emerged at the end of Phase 2 of the project did not represent a final version of the role, but is merely a stage in its ongoing development.

Phase 3 — role evaluation

The aim of this final 3-month phase was to evaluate the role which emerged at the end of Phase 2. This phase consisted of two parts: firstly, of structured interviews with the patients and relatives seen by the ANP to determine their satisfaction with the service provided; and secondly, of questionnaires sent to the healthcare practitioners interviewed during Phase 1 to enquire whether their needs and expectations and those of the service as a whole had been met by the project.

Conclusion

The strategy adopted in this project was based on a Level 4 research methodology which drew heavily on action research and participative techniques, and which saw the outcome of research as being positive change in the situation being investigated rather than the generation of generalisable knowledge and theory. To a large extent, the promise of the action research methodology was realised; not only was a new Advanced Nurse Practitioner role developed and evaluated, but it has also resulted in a noticeable improvement in the provision of care.

In many ways, the methodology of this study is simply a much accelerated example of what happens naturally when any new post is developed. However, because the process took place rapidly under controlled conditions as a funded research project, the end result was a very attractive proposition to healthcare purchasers. The real evaluation of success is the fact that at the end of the project period, funding was taken up jointly by a University and a HealthCare Trust despite severe financial restrictions within both organisations.

References

Glaser, B. and Strauss, A. (1967) *The Discovery of Grounded Theory.* New York: Aldine.

Kolb, D.A. and Fry, R. (1975) Towards an applied theory of experiential learning. In: *The Theories of Group Processes* (C.L. Cooper, ed.) London: John Lilley and Sons.

Schön, D.A. (1983) *The Reflective Practitioner.* London: Temple Smith.

UKCC (1994) *The Future of Professional Practice — the Council's Standards for Education and Practice following Registration.* London: UKCC.

Usher, R. and Bryant, I. (1989) *Adult Education as Theory, Practice and Research.* London: Routledge.

6

Some post-technocratic education projects

Why has educational research been so uneducational? Why hasn't past educational research taught us better educational practice?

William Torbert

We learn by doing and realising what came of what we did

John Dewey

Introduction

The papers in this chapter are drawn mainly from curriculum development work on the Common Foundation Programme for graduates which Melanie Jasper and I carried out over a number of years, and which is referred to in Chapter 3. The first paper provides an outline of the general course philosophy and structure, and the second and third papers expand on two particular aspects of the course.

In the second paper, Melanie describes her work in developing the portfolio workbook as the primary unifying and integrating component of the course, and demonstrates how it is employed to guide the students' study, how it integrates theory and practice, and how it gives meaning to the assessment schedule.

In the third paper, I outline the course evaluation strategy, which is designed as a Level 4 action research project in which the students and teachers attempt to probe the underlying issues of concern in the course. Although this strategy has been employed successfully for some years, no attempt is made in this paper to report on any findings, since, like all Level 4 research, the generalisability of the evaluation lies in the methodology rather than in the findings.

The final paper in this chapter dates back some years and describes an attempt at a patient-centred clinical placement scheme which I implemented whilst working as a staff nurse on 'Ward X'. The experiment was never repeated, and is included partly for historical reasons, but I do believe that, with certain modifications, it could be employed as a powerful method of attitude change in student nurses.

A process-driven common foundation programme for graduates

Melanie Jasper and Gary Rolfe

Introduction

As nursing strives to assert itself as a profession in its own right, nurses are finding that their roles are undergoing a fundamental change from being doctors' handmaidens to becoming autonomous, decision-making managers and clinicians. In the terminology of this book, they are making the transition from nurse–technicians to nurse–practitioners. This changing role requires a similar change in the way that nursing students are educated, and the profession has responded with the introduction of Project 2000, which brought nurse training into the sphere of higher education. It has been argued in this book that, as a technocratic approach to education, Project 2000 is not the most appropriate curriculum model for the education of post-technocratic practitioners, but nevertheless it appears to be here to stay, and all we can do is therefore to construct a framework within the confines of the Project 2000 curriculum that best meets the needs of nurse–practitioners to develop their own personal knowledge and informal theory out of practice.

Project 2000 divided nursing courses into two 18-month parts. Students all follow a Common Foundation Programme (CFP) regardless of their specialism, followed by one of four branch programmes in Adult, Child, Mental Health or Mental Handicap nursing. Provision was also made for nursing students who already possess health-related degrees to follow shortened CFP courses of as little as 6 months duration. One such course is the 9-month shortened CFP for graduates, launched by the University of Portsmouth in January 1991.

During this first intake to the course, which was designed and taught along traditional, technocratic lines, it became increasingly obvious that it was failing to serve the needs of either the students or the curriculum. The reduced timescale (9 months), and the breadth of the material (the whole CFP curriculum),

combined with the pressure to acquire practical skills to a satisfactory standard, resulted in students and staff who were increasingly stressed and failing to achieve the desired outcomes of the
course.

In addition, the students were demotivated by an over-taught
programme which was fragmented and superficial. There was
insufficient time for students to explore subjects to the depth they
required, and their prior knowledge and skills as graduates and
adult learners were not recognised. Furthermore, it is our belief
that many of these criticisms can be directed at Project 2000
courses in general, and that the added pressure of attempting to
complete the CFP in half the prescribed time merely brought the
issues to the fore. It was therefore thought necessary to revise the
course completely in terms of philosophy, teaching and learning
styles and organisation if it was to produce patient-centred nurses
for the future, capable of leading nursing into the next century.

Course philosophy

We have responded to these problems with a course which
seeks to integrate theory and practice by combining a student-
centred approach to learning with theories of reflective practice
within the constraints of a syllabus for professional training. Our
starting point was to examine the educational needs of our
students rather than what knowledge we felt they needed to
acquire, and to ask ourselves the question: '*How* can we teach
these students?', rather than: '*What* should we teach them?'.

This led to the development of a process-driven course, a
course influenced primarily by the learning needs of the student
group rather than by the demands of the syllabus. By process-
driven, we mean that the teaching methods and strategies were
in place before the content, and that the latter was moulded to
fit the former rather than *vice versa*. That is not to say that the
syllabus material is considered to be unimportant. Rather, it is to
give equal importance to how that material is presented, in the
belief that adult students, studying to be professional,
autonomous practitioners, should be educated using methods
which show acknowledgement and respect for their current
status and future role.

Kelly (1989) argued that the development of process-led curricula should begin with a philosophy of education, and in taking the decision as to what methods to employ, we were greatly influenced by the writing of Carl Rogers (1969, 1983) and the andragogical approach of Malcolm Knowles (1984). Rogers' philosophy of student-centred learning derives from the humanistic school of psychology (Maslow, 1968), and argues that human beings have an innate tendency towards growth and development. He suggested that traditional teaching methods stifle this natural growth process, and that the role of the educator (Rogers did not like the word 'teacher') should be to facilitate the learning process in his or her students.

Knowles also addressed the need for facilitation of adult learners in his distinction between pedagogy and andragogy, and this is accomplished by creating a non-threatening environment in which the students are able to participate in their own learning of relevant material. The non-threatening environment is a function of the attitudes of the educator towards her students; participation can be facilitated by employing active group and individual learning methods; and relevance is best ensured by encouraging students to reflect on their own learning needs and to raise them in class. Thus, Rogers eschewed the use of tutor-directed methods such as lecturing, in favour of allowing the students to set both the pace and, to a large extent, the content of the course.

However, our adoption of this approach to education is more than merely an ideological stance; rather, it is a response to the development of the nursing profession with its demands for nurse–practitioners, holistic practice and professional autonomy. We believe that thinking, decision making, problem solving, autonomous nurses will never result from courses where the thinking, decision making, problem solving and autonomy are mainly the responsibility of the course planners and teachers. Autonomous practitioners grow from autonomous students, and autonomous students are students who have a major part to play in what and how they learn.

The principal feature of a student-centred approach to learning is that the students exert a degree of influence over both the content of the course and the methods by which the material will be learnt. However, although student-centred methods have been successfully applied in non-vocational courses, they have been criticised as inappropriate for professional education where prescribed outcomes are expected to be met. We have attempted to address this by providing the students with a list of theoretical and clinical objectives which have to be accomplished, whilst the route to achieving these objectives is individually negotiated by each student.

Course structure

The structure of the course has been designed specifically to facilitate this individualised approach to learning, and takes the form of a reflective spiral curriculum as outlined in Chapter 3. The course includes the following elements:

- A weekly add-on workbook which the students use to achieve both the theoretical and practical objectives. This includes the identification of existing knowledge and skills, action planning for how the week's objectives are to be met, critical incident analysis, reflection on the week's learning and identification of objectives still to be achieved. This component of the course will be outlined in more detail in the following paper.
- Portfolio workshops to actively engage the students in reflecting on practice and theory.
- The use of learning teams both formally and informally to maximise time, knowledge and skill resources.
- Monthly tutorials with the academic tutor to reflect on progress and negotiate the process for achieving the next month's objectives.
- Didactic teaching limited to 1 hour per week.

Thus, although all the students will meet the course objectives for the CFP, they will each plan and negotiate their individual route for achieving them, depending on their prior knowledge and experience, the clinical areas they are based in, and their particular learning needs and wishes.

It is recognised, however, that at first the students will have difficulty in identifying relevant course material and learning needs. Initial content is therefore prescribed, and much of the core syllabus material is covered early in the course. As the students begin to experience clinical situations, they will be encouraged to reflect on those experiences and bring issues and problems arising from them into the classroom to be addressed in a group setting by a variety of interactive teaching methods such as role-play, buzz groups, brainstorming and critical incident work. Course content therefore progresses from being prescribed by the tutor during the initial stages of the course, to becoming more and more student-centred as the course continues. By the end of the course, the students are dictating all the content, based on their clinical needs.

This model has a number of implications for course design which conflict with the traditional higher education model adopted by most Project 2000 course planners. Firstly, the students are introduced into practical clinical placements very early in the course. Rather than equip them with a body of nursing knowledge which they are then expected to apply in practice, the students are facilitated to generate their own knowledge base directly from real-life situations. The emphasis is therefore on 'knowing how' rather than on 'knowing that', and on personal knowledge and informal theory rather than on public, research-based knowledge and formal, generalisable theory.

The course is divided into a number of themes such as 'communication' and 'maintaining a safe environment', each of which lasts for 1 week. Within each theme, the student spends 2 days in a clinical area and 2 days in formal, timetabled study. The theoretical and practical objectives for each week will reflect the theme, and theory and practice are further brought together through the portfolio and workbook. The portfolio is a record of the clinical work undertaken by the student, and includes nursing notes, assessments and other clinical details, while the workbook includes space for a reflective diary and critical incident analysis.

Each week, the timetable includes a keynote lecture which introduces the theme for the week, human relationship skills training, and a case study workshop in which students examine and analyse thematically linked cases through the method of free discussion groups outlined in Chapter 3. This entails exploring a case study individually, then in small groups, and finally as a large group.

For the remaining taught component of the course, the large group is split into small groups of eight, each facilitated by a group tutor. Time is spent in portfolio workshops which provide the students with an opportunity to share their diaries and critical incidents, reflect on their practice and perhaps role-play difficult situations in a warm and supportive learning environment; and in seminar presentations generated from the large group work. The seminars enable the students to identify relevant sources of nursing knowledge, and provides a reliable and time-efficient way of introducing current research-based practice. In keeping with the course structure and philosophy, the seminar programme starts as tutor directed, and progresses to being entirely student-centred by the end of the course, with the students deciding whether the tutor should be present.

Conclusion

This course is a response to the educational requirements of the student nurse–practitioner, and focuses on the identification of learning needs arising directly out of practice and the generation of personal knowledge and informal theory through reflection-on-action. While questioning many of the assumptions of the technocratic higher education model, the course nevertheless attempts to work from inside that model and to develop a post-technocratic reflective spiral curriculum within the constraints of the UKCC guidelines for Project 2000.

Although the graduate-entry CFP has a relatively small intake, the course framework could be effectively utilised with larger group numbers, and as there is a gradual transition within the course from tutor-led to student-centred activity, we are currently looking at ways in which tutor input can be decreased. These include a greater focus on individual learning contracts and the use of student-facilitated seminar and small group work, and it is envisaged that these measures will allow for increased student–staff ratios. However, a slight note of caution must be sounded, since although large intakes might be economically desirable, we need to recognise the different nature of the learning outcomes required of a professional course compared to non-vocational education.

Whereas non-vocational courses are concerned primarily with cognitive objectives, in professional education equal attention must be given to the skills and affective domains (Jarvis, 1983). Skills and attitudes are best addressed through a variety of small group techniques such as role-play, T-groups, games and simulations, and whereas some of these activities lend themselves to larger student numbers, most are best conducted in groups of ten of less. Thus, although the student–staff ratio might be increased by the introduction of learning contracts and tutorless seminars, there will always be some areas in any professional course which will require intensive tutor input.

The aim of this paper has been to describe a common foundation course for postgraduate students based on the reflective spiral curriculum discussed in Chapter 3. Our starting point was with the needs of the students rather than the demands of the syllabus, and in this way we feel we have designed a framework which has not only accommodated our beliefs in student-centred learning, but also the demands of a curriculum for post-technocratic professional education. The course aims to facilitate student choice, control and responsibility for their own learning and for their clinical practice, which entails a major shift in attitude for students and tutors alike. Although the focus of this paper has been on a shortened CFP for graduates, we believe that the framework has universal application, and could be effectively adapted to any professional training course where the aim is to bring together theory and practice and produce competent, autonomous practitioners capable of lifelong learning.

References

Jarvis, P. (1983) *Professional Education*. London: Croom Helm.

Kelly, A.V. (1989) *The Curriculum: Theory and Practice*, 3rd edn. London: Paul Chapman.

Knowles, M. (1984) *The Adult Learner, a Neglected Species*. Houston: Gulf.

Maslow A.H. (1968) *Towards a Psychology of Being*, 2nd edn. New York: Van Nostrand Reinhold.

Rogers C.R. (1969) *Freedom to Learn*. Columbus: Merrill.

Rogers C.R. (1983) *Freedom to Learn for the 80s*. Columbus: Merrill.

The portfolio workbook as a strategy for student-centred learning

Melanie Jasper

Introduction

The use of action research in evaluation and development enables courses to respond rapidly to student needs. One such strategy to evolve in the course described in the previous paper is the creation of a portfolio type workbook which provides the students with the framework and components of the course, but enables them to select the learning strategies by which they achieve them. The workbook has been tested and evaluated over the past 4 years by the teachers, students and practitioners, and has been developed during that time into the integrating mechanism for the course. It has been pivotal in enabling the students to devise strategies to rationalise the theory–practice interface, whilst at the same time providing a method of assessment which enables the teachers to monitor the students' progress on a monthly basis. This paper describes the current structure and use of the workbook, and addresses issues such as assessment and ethical concerns. However, as with all components of the course, it is dynamic and changing constantly in response to student and course demands.

The overall evaluation at the end of the first year of the course (1992) was extremely positive. However, the students identified the need for clearer direction in terms of learning outcomes that they could use to structure their work (Jasper, 1994). Initially, the structure of the portfolio had been the decision of each student in consultation with their academic tutor. This proved to be insufficient in enabling the student to select learning outcomes and needs and focus these on the time and resources available for the week. This led to the design of a portfolio workbook which guides the student on a weekly basis through the course content.

This content is organised around a weekly theme, such as Communication or Loss and Bereavement, which identifies the theoretical and practical components for the week. The workbook combines the strategies of reflection on prior knowledge and experience with active identification of learning needs to enable the students to plan their time to maximum effect. The students identify learning objectives, both clinical and theoretical, and plan how these will be met throughout the week. In addition, a critical incident analysis is completed weekly and used in the portfolio workshop, and a reflective diary of the week's work summarises progress and further learning needs, thus completing the reflective cycle. The components of the workbook are discussed more fully below.

Components of the workbook

The components of the workbook can be summarised as:

1. essential reading, clinical and theoretical objectives relating to the week's theme;
2. identification of prior learning and experience;
3. identification of additional learning needed to achieve objectives;
4. strategies to achieve these, with checklist;
5. critical incident analysis;
6. reflective journal detailing the week's achievements and experiences.

Essential reading, clinical and theoretical objectives

These are identified for the students by the teacher leading the theme. The students have to achieve the same learning outcomes as those following the 18-month CFP, but in a third of the time. Hence, maximum use is made of the prior learning skills of the graduates, such as effective reading and note-taking. Students are guided to key texts and expected to pre-read these prior to the start of the week's theme. The theoretical objectives provide the level of knowledge to be achieved and thus enable the students to gauge their own workload needs. The clinical objectives are identified by theme in CFP documentation, which is given to the students at the beginning of the course to enable them to gain an overall appreciation of the skills they need to achieve. By attaching these objectives to the weekly theme, they become manageable both to the student and to the clinical practice supervisor and act as a mechanism for organising practical experiences.

Identification of prior learning and experience

The graduate students are at least 5 years older than the majority of the standard entry students, and bring to the course a variety of study, work and life experiences. These are acknowledged as foundational to the course, as they provide the starting point for each individual student to plan to achieve the objectives. The students assess these previous experiences and achievements against the weekly objectives and identify those yet to be met.

Identification of additional learning needed to achieve the objectives

In turn, the students make most effective use of this prior knowledge by identifying areas of the course where they need to concentrate their time and energy in order to meet the specified learning outcomes. Many choose not to attend the optional life, behavioural and social science programmes, because these have been covered at a higher level in their first degrees, preferring instead to work on nursing theory.

Strategies to achieve learning objectives

An action plan for learning arises from the objectives identified by the student. Individual skills are entered into a grid which asks the student to record the development of these skills on an incremental basis (Table 6.1).

This action plan also enables the supervisor of clinical practice to work with the student to plan the most appropriate experi-

Table 6.1 An example of an action plan

Objective	Date of achievement				
	A	B	C	D	E
1 Give an injection					
2 Administer tablets					
3 Measure medicines					
and so on, where:					
A - not yet encountered					
B - observed					
C - undertaken under supervision					
D - undertaken alone					
E - competence achieved					

ence to meet the specified objectives. Thus, the student has a mechanism for self-assessment throughout the course in terms of achieving the objectives, and the supervisor can also use the action plan to monitor progress. The action plan is used in conjunction with the summative clinical placement form to provide evidence of skills acquisition.

It is, of course, impossible to guarantee that the student will encounter every situation or skill required during the week of that particular theme. Therefore the action plan becomes part of the ongoing review process between the supervisor, teacher and student in order to ensure the development and competence of the required skills.

Critical incident analysis

Each week the student analyses a critical incident relating to the week's theme. This is subsequently used in learning team work at the weekly portfolio workshop. The emphasis for this component is placed on an incident that is significant for the student in terms of his learning, and it provides the material for examining the relationship between theory and practice. It also serves the important purpose of identifying areas that the student finds stressful, providing the indication for extra work related to the theme, or increased tutorial support.

Reflective element

This is the culmination of the week's work and focuses the students on their achievements in relation to the theme, and to the learning outcomes of the course in general. The students are asked to review their week, identify the objectives that have been achieved, and those that are yet to be acquired. By reviewing their progress on a regular basis the students gain the satisfaction of monitoring and controlling their own learning.

The latter two components of the workbook draw together the educational theories of critical incident analysis (Flanagan, 1954; Smith and Russell, 1991) and reflective practice (Boyd and Fales, 1983; Schön, 1991). These have their roots in the theories of experiential learning (Kolb, 1984), suggesting that a valid way of learning is by systematically examining experiences through deconstruction and subsequent reconstruction in terms of what has been learnt in order to develop strategies for future use. By the end of each week the student has a clear picture of the learning that has occurred, and what more needs to be done to achieve the learning objectives.

All of the workbook strategies are student-directed, and key into the natural motivation of the student to learn (Rogers, 1983) by enabling him to acknowledge his previous learning and build on this to achieve externally identified criteria. They also enable the student to take control of his learning and respect the student's capacity to take responsibility as an adult to identify and fulfil his learning needs (Knowles, 1984). Although this sounds deceptively simple in itself, the infrastructure needed to support this type of learning and the development in terms of teachers and students attitudes are complex.

Evaluation at the end of the second year, that is, after the workbook structure had been used for a year, suggested that the reflective cycle inherent within the structure had been successful. The students now 'knew what they had to know' and had the confidence that they were building on previously acquired skills. In addition, their time management had improved as they were identifying key areas of knowledge and skill to concentrate on. The development of reflective skills was evident in the rate at which students were able to relate theory to practice and to espouse theories built up through custom and practice. Not only was there evidence of initial learning, it was quite clear that the students were practising reflexively as experiential learning occurred. However, whilst the structure of the workbook seemed to be effective, it was clear that attention needed to be paid to the role of the teacher at this time.

The teacher's role

The philosophy of student-centred learning requires the espousal of an alternative value system on the part of the teachers in order to enable the students to take responsibility for their own learning (Rogers, 1983). This is a radical shift from the teacher-centred philosophy which underpins most nurse teaching. For the workbook to be effective, teachers need to facilitate and motivate students to structure their time effectively, and to help students identify the mechanisms by which they can achieve objectives. Throughout this course the student works closely with an academic tutor on a one-to-one basis, meeting at least monthly. In addition, the teacher works with a learning team of 6–8 students for all parts of the course that involve small group work. In this way the student–teacher relationship builds into a supportive one, where any problems can be identified and resolved quickly and effectively. This represents a move away from the largely didactic teaching methods traditionally employed in nurse education, and requires a re-orientation of both attitudes and behaviour by the teacher.

The student too is, to some extent, faced with a type of learning that is different to their expectations. This self-directed methodology depends for its success on the maturity of the students and their capacity to take responsibility for their learning in terms of organising their time and achieving their objectives. Different students need varying amounts of support in this. However, it has been found that although the initial weeks of the course are very intensive in terms of time given to students, this quickly decreases as the students become more independent and shed their preconceived ideas of the nature of education from their previous experience.

The workbook is also of benefit to clinical supervisors in that students have predetermined objectives each week which guide practical experience, thus reducing the time needed for organisation and direction. By using the workbook as the underpinning for all work, the supervisor has a record of experiences and skills gained on a continual basis. This facilitates feedback, with the final assessment becoming a technical device rather than the emotive instrument of previous years.

Assessment of the portfolio workbook

The portfolio workbook contributes to both the formative and summative assessment schedules of the course. The dichotomy between ongoing development and terminal assessment is managed by the active recognition of the two as separate processes, with the former as developmental and the latter as evaluative.

Formative assessment

Used formatively, the workbook enables the learning needs of the student to be identified, the acquisition of learning objectives monitored, and the progress of the student to be continuously assessed. This is achieved through regular tutorial contact, at least on a monthly basis, between the student and academic tutor; and through the supervisory relationship between student and clinician in practice placements. The workbook provides the point of discussion through which the previous learning is reviewed and future learning is planned. This strategy has the additional benefit of encouraging a supportive and nurturing relationship to develop between tutor and student and between clinician and student, which facilitates the early identification of problems and eases the task of summative assessment.

Summative assessment

The portfolio, together with an examination which makes use of its content (Rolfe, 1993), forms the summative assessment for the course. During the last 6 weeks of the course the student builds a 'model' client profile in the portfolio by relating the themes to one particular client. This model client is then used as the base material for the examination questions. All students answer the same two questions in the examination (relating to behavioural and life sciences, and to nursing process) but in relation to their particular client. Thus the principle of individual student relevance is maintained (see Chapter 3).

In addition the portfolio is assessed as a separate piece of work. Portfolios in professional education tend to be used formatively rather than summatively (Budnick and Beaver, 1984; Lambeth *et al.*, 1989; Oeschle *et al.*, 1990), with the result that there is a sparsity of information relating to criteria for portfolio assessment. The major problem in assessing work of this kind is its individual nature; thus it is not amenable to standardisation in terms of normative content. As the portfolio is part of the Diploma of Higher Education (with the CFP component discounted for the grade of the final award), it was originally ungraded other than to make the distinction between pass and fail, in recognition of previously identified problems relating to portfolio type assessments (Glen and Hight, 1992; Gerrish, 1993). A pass grade was awarded to students who completed the portfolio requirements as identified in the students' guidelines (Table 6.2).

The portfolios were moderated by a tutor panel to ensure that the close relationship between student and tutor did not interfere with the assessment process, and to act as a developmental

Table 6.2 Student guidelines for the portfolio

Objectives of the portfolio

In compiling the portfolio you will:

a) Study in detail at least one aspect of care in relation to one patient that you have nursed each week.
b) If appropriate, i.e if an area of care is being examined, write a care plan for that client with reference to that aspect of care, and supported by researched material.
c) Critique and evaluate the care being received by the client.
d) Reflect on your own actions and contribution to nursing care, with the aim of identifying knowledge and skill deficits, and planning to remedy these.

Each week's work should be clearly delineated in order to facilitate the marking of the portfolio.

Table 6.3 Portfolio marking criteria at level 2

Criteria

1	There is a clear focus on an aspect of care for each entry.
2	Evidence is provided of integration of subjects which inform nursing practice.
3	There is evidence of reflective practice through a systematic and logical evaluation of the aspect of care.
4	The student demonstrates the ability to assess, plan and evaluate nursing care.
5	The portfolio incorporates relevant usage of literature in an attempt to rationalise and support conclusions reached.
6	There is evidence of professional development by justifying conclusions reached.
7	There is evidence of ability to self-direct personal and professional development.
8	The portfolio demonstrates an ability to identify own learning and learning needs demonstrated by critical incident analysis.
9	The portfolio demonstrates acquisition of nursing knowledge through the integration of course components.
10	It is a logical and sequential portfolio, referenced where necessary to an accepted format.

Each criterion is awarded marks according to the following scale:

0–3	little or no evidence of satisfying any aspect of the criterion.
4	some evidence of satisfying at least one aspect of the criterion.
5	evidence of more aspects of the criterion being satisfied.
6	evidence of nearly all aspects of the criterion being satisfied.
7–10	evidence of the criterion being met in all its aspects.

exercise for other members of teaching staff. However, the standard of work generated by the students was so high that the course team asked the Board of Examiners to award distinction grades to some students. This was based on the quality of the reflective process evidenced in the portfolios, and the identification of the developmental processes undergone by the students. This provided the stimulus for the teachers to develop a more sophisticated method of identifying students achieving distinction level work with the addition of specific criterion-referenced marking guidelines (Table 6.3).

The strategy of providing the students with clear guidelines for the assessment at the beginning of the course enables them to plan their work to meet these criteria and moves the locus of control over the process further towards the students. The marking criteria are sufficiently broad to encompass the individuality of each student whilst ensuring a uniform standard is met.

Although by the end of the course the very size and content of the portfolio makes the marking onerous, the task is made easier by the structured format and the fact that the tutor has seen it on a regular basis throughout the course. It is the intention of the course team to develop further marking criteria and a way of recording the ongoing assessment on a formal basis to facilitate the summative evaluation.

Evaluation of the portfolio workbook

Minor modifications to the layout of the book were the only changes to the format, and all students found it easy to use, logical in format, and central to the management of their learning. This has remained the structure for the last 2 years, and looks unlikely to change.

The teachers and clinical supervisors were overwhelmingly positive in relation to the expected outcomes of using the portfolio. It eased the recording of continuous assessment, and provided a more detailed picture of the students learning than had previously been possible. It also enabled assessment of the degree to which the students were able to relate theory to practice, and to generate theory from practice in a reflective cycle, a type of learning difficult to assess using conventional methods. Teachers appreciated the focus that the portfolio workbook brought to tutorial time, as specific areas of discussion arose from reviewing the work demonstrated in the workbook.

Ethical issues

The summative use of assessment raises many issues in terms of objectivity, reliability and standardisation in comparison to more traditional methods of assessment. It can be argued that the only objectivity required in relation to the portfolio is that of the marker in assessing its content as evidence of the required acquisition of competence. The relationship between the tutor and student during the portfolio process is necessarily close, involving the development of trust to enable the student to share his experiences honestly and to facilitate learning from those experiences. There is a potential dilemma for the tutor in that relationship if the student does not achieve the required standard, but this can be overcome by the internal moderation of all portfolios.

How can the reliability of portfolios be assessed? Whilst the portfolio cannot test the knowledge possessed by the student, it can provide evidence of the application of it to practice. Similarly, the cognitive and affective elements of the educational process can be documented, providing some evidence of the acquisition of 'institutionally approved' attitudes and movement towards a professional ethos. However, the value of the portfolio workbook lies in the nature of the process rather than the end product *per se*. The workbook itself merely documents the process, rather than supplying any measure of quality. Quality and standards of practice need to be verified in another way, in this case by a practice assessment document, and the sufficiency of the knowledge-base can be tested by an examination.

Discussion

The portfolio workbook is an innovative attempt to enable the different knowledge-bases of theory and practice to be bridged. It acts as the organising factor for learning nursing by simultaneously guiding the students to what they need to know as competent practitioners, that is, the theory underpinning practice in the reality of their clinical placement. Combined with reflective workshops, case-study work and seminar presentations, the workbook enables the students to rationalise the theory–practice gap, and provides an essential mechanism for dealing with stress engendered by the difference between personal and public value systems.

Whilst the workbook has validated our underlying philosophy about education, the biggest gain has been in the way that students have moved from teacher-dependency to self-direction. In terms of preparing nurses to work in a changing health service, and to demonstrate their worth in economic terms, this is more than just an ideological stance. As Jasper and Rolfe (1993) wrote:

> We believe that thinking, decision-making, problem-solving, autonomous nurses will never result from courses where the thinking, decision-making, problem-solving and autonomy are mainly the responsibility of the course planners and teachers. Autonomous practitioners grow from autonomous students, and autonomous students are students who have a major part in what and how they learn.

The students, therefore, are our best advertisement for the success of the portfolio workbook, in that they have produced a quality of work which exemplifies the development of autonomous practitioners. Many have commented that they wished they could have used this type of strategy before because it enables theory and practice to 'make sense' so much more quickly. Whilst all have moved into branch studies following the CFP which involves a different type of portfolio compilation, several have commented on the foundational basis of the CFP portfolio workbook in terms of how it helped them 'learn how to learn'.

It has been an honour to have worked with the graduate students, and it is acknowledged that these may be a special group in terms of student-centred learning strategies. However, there seems to be no reason why this strategy should not be incorporated into all forms of education and training where there is both a practical and theoretical element. It is my belief that the academic level of the students is irrelevant to the use of a workbook strategy. What is essential is the capacity of the teachers to embrace the underlying philosophy and abandon teacher-centred methods of education. The re-write of the Project 2000 course has incorporated the workbook and other strategies from the shortened course for graduates, in the belief that student-centred strategies can also be used in the management of learning for large intakes of students. Alongside this will run a concurrent programme of teacher development to enable maximum use to be made of the radically different strategies for nurse education envisaged for the future. The strategy of the portfolio workbook is constantly monitored and improved in response to students and teachers evaluations, ensuring that the quality of education in nurse training is maintained whilst at the same time developing innovative mechanisms to achieve this standard.

References

Boyd, E.M. and Fales, A.W. (1983) Reflective learning: key to learning from experience. *J. Hum. Psychol.*, **23**, 2, 99–117.

Budnick, D. and Beaver, S. (1984) A student perspective on the portfolio. *Nursing Outlook*, **32**, 5, 268–269.

Flanagan, J. (1954) The critical incident technique. *Psychol. Bull.*, **51**, 327–358.

Gerrish, K. (1993) An evaluation of a portfolio as an assessment tool for teaching practice placements. *Nurse Education Today*, **13**, 172–179.

Glen, S. and Hight, N. (1992) Portfolios: an affective assessment strategy? *Nurse Education Today*, **12**, 416–423.

Jasper, M. and Rolfe, G. (1993) A framework for a process-driven Common Foundation Programme for graduates. *Int. J. Nursing Stud.*, **30**, 5, 377–385.

Jasper, M. (1994) A shortened common foundation programme for graduates — the students' experience of student-centred learning. *Nurse Education Today*, **14**, 238–244.

Knowles, M. (1984) *The Adult Learner, a Neglected Species*. Houston: Gulf.

Kolb, D.A. (1984) *Experiential Learning*. New Jersey: Prentice-Hall.

Lambeth, S.O., Volden, C.M. and Oeschle, L.H. (1989) Portfolios: they work for RNs. *J. Nursing Education*, **28**, 1, 42–44.

Oeschle, L.H., Volden, C.M. and Lambeth, S.O. (1990) Portfolios and RNs: an evaluation. *J. Nursing Education*, **29**, 2, 540–559.

Rogers, C.R. (1983) *Freedom to learn for the '80s*. Ohio: Merrill.

Rolfe, G. (1993) Towards a theory of student–centred nurse education: overcoming the constraints of a professional curriculum. *Nurse Education Today*, **13**, 149–154.

Schön, D. (1991) *The Reflective Practitioner*. San Francisco: Jossey-Bass.

Smith, A. and Russell, J. (1991) Using critical learning incidents in nurse education. *Nurse Education Today*, **11**, 285–291.

Listening to students: course evaluation as action research

Gary Rolfe

Introduction

The aim of this research project was to evaluate a Common Foundation Programme (CFP) in nursing run by Melanie Jasper and myself, which was described earlier in this chapter. What was required was an indication of the students' feelings about being on the course; that is, a measure of process rather than outcome, and of course structure and learning methods rather than content, since the latter were already being assessed in a number of other ways. The course was designed along student-centred lines, with course members participating in content and process decisions, and we wanted the evaluation to reflect the same philosophy.

Unfortunately, our previous experience of course evaluation, both as students and teachers, has been generally disappointing. Most evaluations utilise tools generated by the teacher, which effectively ignore the students' agenda. The information generated is often of little practical use, with the focus being either too general or too specific, and students are usually not briefed to write constructive and useful criticism.

Furthermore, response rates are often disappointingly low, reflecting both a lack of ownership of the findings, and the belief that whatever feedback the students give will not be acted upon. And since evaluations usually occur at the end of courses, students often feel that even if action is taken, it will be too late to be of benefit to them. This often results in a 'see-saw' effect in which changes suggested by one intake to the course are reversed by the following group. In short, our experience of course evaluation has been of an unthinking ritual with little commitment by the teachers to act on the information generated.

In attempting to rectify some of these problems, the research project adopted several principles:

- Evaluation should be an ongoing, integral part of a course, and not just a retrospective exercise.
- Curriculum planning should likewise continue throughout, based on findings from regular evaluation sessions. In this way, the course will retain its flexibility and respond to the needs of the students.
- The students should play an active role in the process of evaluation. Course evaluation is part of the education process, and the students can learn and practice high level cognitive skills through participation in the evaluation of their course.
- All evaluation is by definition subjective, so there is little point in searching for objective methods or bringing in outside evaluators. Rather, we should embrace the subjectivity of the evaluation process and collect a variety of perceptions of the course, not just those prescribed by the teacher.

Clearly, the above principles lend themselves perfectly to a Level 4 participative action research approach in which:

> all those involved contribute both to the creative thinking that goes into the enterprise — deciding on what is to be looked at, the methods of inquiry, and making sense of what is found out — and also contribute to the action which is the subject of the research. (Reason, 1988)

This approach implies not only that the 'subjects' of the research play an active part in every stage of the project, but that the findings are immediately acted upon, thereby bringing about direct change in the organisation or process under investigation.

Thus, the students were seen as equal partners in, and joint owners of, the project, with the intention that the material generated should be of direct benefit to the people who provided it. It was therefore considered important that evaluation should start at the beginning of the course, with immediate application of the findings.

The role of the teacher in the early stage of the evaluation was that of enabling the students by constructing a framework in which the process could evolve. In psychological terms, this involved adopting an attitude of permissiveness and non-judgementalism, acknowledging the importance of the evaluation, and ensuring that the students understood its purpose. In practical terms, it required the provision of space in the timetable for the evaluation to take place, and ensuring that the students had the necessary research skills for the task.

An overview of the evaluation process

An initial meeting with the students was called in order to engage them in the project and to present the philosophy of participative research. In the second meeting, the students divided into small groups of four or five to pursue specific areas of the evaluation. Students were given a completely free hand to choose which aspects of the course to evaluate and the methods they would employ. In allowing the students this freedom, we made the assumption that they would choose issues that had personal meaning, importance and significance to them, and that they would therefore invest high emotional energy in their chosen areas. We might expect, then, that their evaluations would be highly subjective, even biased, despite their best efforts at objectivity. However, this is seen as an advantage, since their findings will reflect issues of relevance to them as individuals.

At this stage, the research strategy split into two parallel streams. The students proceeded to investigate their chosen aspects of the course in five small groups, examining areas such as the effectiveness of self-directed learning, communication, and the use of group work. All five groups chose to use questionnaires to collect their data, the main reasons being those of speed and simplicity, although a wide range of methods was open to them.

The material generated by the questionnaires provided a rich source of information about the issues that were relevant and important to the students, but it is by definition surface information, reflecting their immediate perceived needs. The course teachers held a philosophy of group dynamics based on the work of Bion (1961), who argued that as well as a surface agenda aimed at meeting their stated needs, in this case the need for education, all groups also have a deep and usually unconscious agenda of which their members might be totally unaware.

Therefore, at the same time that the students were administering their questionnaires, the course teachers were attempting to probe the deeper group issues by analysing and deconstructing the research instruments. This involved trying to get underneath the surface meaning of the questions to look for deeper motivations. It is recognised that what this produces is a subjective impression by the teachers of what the unconscious group issues might be, and therefore this analysis was then used to construct an interview schedule for a depth interview with each group in order to test out the teachers' hypotheses, and to attempt to bring the unconscious group agenda into the conscious awareness of the group members. A flow chart of the full research process is shown in Figure 6.1.

This process, although time consuming, generated a very rich fund of information about all aspects of the course. On the one hand, we had the information collected by the students themselves concerning the issues which they saw as important, and which they wanted addressing in time to benefit them on their course. On the other hand, we hopefully gained access to the hidden agenda of the group, to the feelings, attitudes and anxieties of the course members based on the material from the group interviews.

The final task of the teachers and students was to integrate the findings from the students' inquiry with the material from the interviews into a broad and holistic evaluation of the course, and to negotiate ways of acting on the students' recommendations while at the same time addressing their feelings and anxieties.

This can raise problems, since the two agendas often appear to conflict. For example, many of the students on the course were having difficulty in setting their own objectives and directing their own study, and this was reflected in their evaluation by a request for a return to more formal teaching methods. However, the group interviews uncovered a great deal of anxiety about the examination at the end of the course and the depth of knowledge required to pass it. What emerged was that it was not the process of self-directed study that was causing difficulty, but a perceived lack of information and guidance about the content and format of the exam, which was resolved very simply by providing information and reassurance.

This was a very different intervention from that originally requested by the students, and it demonstrates the advantages of probing beyond their surface agenda. According to Bion's theory

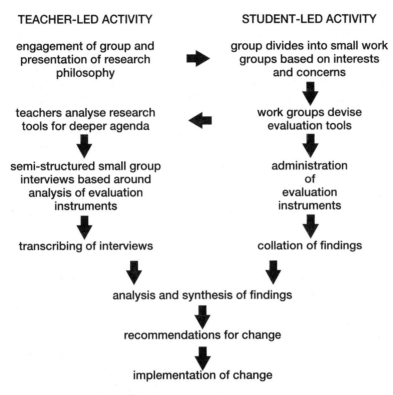

Figure 6.1 A flow chart of the research process

of group dynamics, the tension created by the deep agenda of exam anxiety was translated into a 'fight or flight' response in which blame was placed on the nearest and most convenient peg, in this case the issue of self-directed study. Had we simply responded to the students' request for a return to a more formal curriculum, the real cause of their anxiety would not have been addressed, and would inevitably have been resurrected by the next intake of students, who would probably have blamed it on something quite different. The see-saw effect is therefore eliminated by getting to the real source of student discontent rather than accepting their criticism at face value.

Validity of the framework

The issue of validity raises the question of whether an instrument measures what it claims, in this case, the thoughts and feelings of the students about issues of course process and learning methods. This is a complex and difficult area that cannot be fully addressed here, but we must be careful not to confuse the validity of the research framework with the validity of the individual instruments generated from that framework, although the two issues are, of course, linked.

It could be argued that the instruments devised by the students will not have been tested for validity, and that therefore the information they yield will be of limited value. Nevertheless, they will reflect areas of concern and importance to the students, and we would therefore maintain that, whatever instruments they construct, the framework will be valid in that it highlights areas that are relevant for that particular student group. Furthermore, the weaknesses and biases in the construction of the instruments will give an indication of particular issues of concern within those areas to be picked up in the group interviews.

For example, one group of students chose to look at the issue of self-directed learning. We would argue that in making that choice, the students indicated that self-directed learning was a particularly relevant issue to them, and this assumption was later borne out in the group interview. Furthermore, the students' questionnaire contained several leading questions and was, by conventional standards, poorly designed. Nevertheless, an analysis of the content and intention of those questions highlighted possible issues of concern within the area of self-directed learning, and again these leads were followed up during the interview. This revealed that the students had believed their questionnaire to be fair and bias-free, and they were genuinely surprised that we had managed to uncover specific problem areas which would otherwise have gone unnoticed.

Thus, although the student-generated tools within the evaluation framework will almost certainly lack validity, their purpose is to raise issues of importance as much as to collect data, and they are therefore to some extent a means to an end. However, we would argue that the overall framework *can* be said to be valid in that it uncovers areas of concern, it is a vehicle for the students to express their thoughts and feelings about course structure and process issues, and it can provide a forum to address deep issues which might be acting as a block to learning.

Conclusion

This paper has outlined a strategy for a student-centred approach to course evaluation drawing on collaborative inquiry and action research techniques. Although specifically designed for a CFP in nursing, we believe that this method is applicable to any course in further or higher education. It requires a reappraisal of outmoded and redundant notions about the role of evaluation within educational courses, and has, we believe, several advantages over traditional methods. Firstly, it gets below the surface issues and highlights the underlying causes of problems and difficulties; secondly, teachers and students are made aware of issues of importance which might interfere with the process of learning *as they arise*; thirdly, students are put in touch with, and are therefore more able to deal with, their own feelings and anxieties about the course; and fourthly, it could help to develop analytical skills and high level cognitive functioning in the students.

On the negative side, an evaluation of this kind can be extremely threatening to teachers, since it involves a loss of control over the evaluation process, a result of which is that they are left exposed to criticism by the students. It also demands a prerequisite attitude of student-centredness in the course teacher, and a great deal of commitment to look critically at both their course and their teaching. Finally, it might appear to be an extremely time consuming approach to evaluation, but in fact it need take only about one hour per week, and in our experience, this has been well spent time which has contributed greatly to the ongoing development of our course.

References

Bion, W.R. (1961) *Experiences in Groups*. London: Routledge.
Reason, P. (1988) *Human Inquiry in Action*. London: Sage.

The Ward X experiment: a patient-centred clinical placement

Gary Rolfe

Introduction

Throughout this book, a great deal of emphasis has been placed on the importance of the individual therapeutic relationship between the nurse–practitioner and her patient as the primary means of generating informal theory out of practice. However, the focus has been entirely on the nurse's side of the equation, on the importance of reflecting on what it is like to be a nurse in this therapeutic relationship, and it might be useful when constructing an informal theory about a particular clinical situation to also have some personal knowledge and paradigm cases of how it might feel to be a patient in that situation.

Carl Rogers wrote of the importance of empathy in the therapeutic relationship, of being able 'to sense the client's private world as if it were your own, but without ever losing the "as if" quality' (Rogers, 1957), but this component of education has been largely overlooked by curriculum writers. Furthermore, it appears that rather than redress the balance, post-technocratic education might even make the situation worse by emphasising the practicum as a place for professional development and theory construction.

The traditional approach to helping the nurse to understand what it is like to be a patient has been to employ classroom methods such as role-play, psychodrama, discussions, simulations and group process activities such as T-groups. However, it can be seen that this is very much a technocratic solution in which formal theory is employed to direct and shape the experiences of the student.

It could be argued that a truly patient-centred approach to nurse education should be based on two premises that run counter to the above model. Firstly, that we should be learning *from* the patient rather than learning *about* the patient, and that therefore the patient is the real expert; and secondly, that the use of role-play, simulations and group experiences should be patient-centred rather than nurse-centred. That is, they should be role-plays and simulations of the experience of being a patient rather than of being a nurse, and in a setting which is as close to the therapeutic environment as possible, preferably in the therapeutic environment itself. It can be seen that this approach combines the participative teaching methods of classroom based education with the real-life clinical setting in which the student plays or simulates the role of a patient in a working clinical environment, preferably over an extended period.

Some precedents

Neither role-play nor simulations are new or even recent educational techniques. Role-play is a tried and tested method in the repertoire of most teachers, and is often employed in training nurses to interact therapeutically with patients. Simulators of one kind or another have been used in industry and the armed forces since the 1940s, usually because of the high cost or the dangers and difficulties involved in training personnel with real equipment. Davies (1971) defined a simulator as designed to represent a real situation, to provide a student with controls over that situation, and to vary conditions during training, so that the task can be made progressively more difficult.

Some examples of this specialised form of role-play are the war games and exercises used by the army, business games such as 'In Basket', and the computer aided aircraft simulations used in training pilots. In nurse education, clinical situations are sometimes simulated so the student can practice ward management. However, the focus in both role-play and simulations is almost always on the nurse, and although the role of the patient is played out, it is usually as part of the supporting cast, and the experiences gained from playing the role are rarely examined and learnt from. Additionally, the playing-out of the situation in a safe environment is at the same time the attraction of role-play and also its greatest limitation, since an element of danger and risk-taking adds to the realism of the situation and heightens its emotional impact. The difference between a simulation in a classroom and in a real clinical setting is the difference between a battle exercise using blanks and one using live ammunition.

Two well-documented examples of intensive simulations from outside of nursing are worth considering, since they highlight not only the intensity of the emotional experience that can be gained from a well-constructed, realistic simulation, but also the inherent dangers that are the potential cost of that realism. The first example, a 'behavioural study of obedience' (Milgram, 1963) had people playing the role of 'experimenter' by administering electric shocks to a 'subject' in a 'learning experiment'. Unknown to them, the 'subject' was really an actor, and the 'experimenters' were themselves the subjects. To Milgram's surprise, all 40 subjects administered what they thought were electric shocks of 300 volts to the 'victim', at which point he began kicking on the wall and screaming. Equally disturbing was the effect on the subjects themselves. Milgram describes the behaviour of one of the subjects, a businessman, who administered 'shocks' of what he thought to be 400 volts to the victim:

> Within 20 minutes he was reduced to a twitching, stuttering wreck, who was rapidly approaching a point of nervous collapse. He constantly pulled on his earlobe, and twisted his hands. At one point he pushed his fist into his forehead and muttered: 'Oh God, let's stop it'. And yet he continued to respond to every word of the experimenter, and obeyed to the end. (Milgram, 1963)

This experiment raises many ethical questions, particularly in the way that the subjects were deceived into believing that they were administering real electric shocks. Nevertheless, it highlights how people will continue to play the role given to them, despite intense discomfort, and emphasises the need for a clearly stated and constantly available opt-out clause in any training programme involving role-play.

In a similar experiment, although without the deception of the former, Zimbardo (1972) assigned student volunteers the roles of either 'prisoner' or 'jailer' in a mock prison in the cellars of Stanford University. The experiment was supposed to last for 2 weeks, but:

> The prison situation transformed most of the subjects who played the role of 'guards' into brutal sadists and most of those who played the role of 'prisoners' into abject, frightened, and submissive men, some having such severe mental symptoms that they had to be released after a few days. In fact, the reactions of both groups were so intense that the exper-

iment which was to have lasted for two weeks was broken off after six days. (Fromm, 1973)

This clearly demonstrates the emotional intensity generated by an extended role-play in a realistic setting, since it is unlikely that the experiment would have had the same impact if played out in a classroom over a much shorter period of time. It also serves to highlight once again that along with greater realism and greater emotional commitment by the students, comes a greater risk of danger.

Probably the most useful precedent is the therapeutic community. The term was first used by Tom Main in 1946 to describe his work with demoralised soldiers suffering from battle fatigue during the Second World War. The main exponent of this form of treatment is Maxwell Jones, who began working with ex-prisoners of war, and later founded the Henderson Hospital which treats people suffering from sociopathic disorders. The prospectus for the Henderson sums up the method of treatment as follows:

> At the Henderson the patients participate with staff in a living-and-learning situation throughout the 24 hours. This shared responsibility involves staff and patients together in administrative, policy and management decisions as far as is appropriate and realistic. It does not mean that 'the patient runs the show' but it does mean that the patients who live throughout the 24 hours with their fellows and assist in the management of crises and problems have a say in who is admitted and when someone is discharged.

The nature of the therapeutic community is such that there is little distinction between learning and teaching on the one hand, and therapy on the other, and also between staff learning and teaching and patient learning and teaching. However, Jones suggests that the formal teaching of student nurses should still take place within all-staff settings, albeit in unstructured and multidisciplinary sensitivity groups.

The Ward X experiment

The Ward X experiment gave student psychiatric nurses the opportunity to take part in a simulation exercise of role-playing a patient. The role-play took place over a period of 6 weeks in a clinical environment which will be referred to as Ward X, in the company of other, 'real' patients. The students entered as fully as possible into the patient lifestyle, not only socialising and eating with the other patients, but participating in group therapy and sleeping some nights in the patients' dormitory.

Ward X was an Alcohol Treatment Unit in the grounds of a typical Victorian psychiatric hospital. It was staffed entirely by psychiatric nurses and students came to the unit in the final year of their training for a 12-week placement. The course of therapy undergone by alcoholics in the clinic consisted of 6 weeks of intensive group work as residents. One of the reasons that a residential programme was thought to be necessary was because treatment carried on outside of formal group therapy, and the environment of the unit was considered to be therapeutic in itself.

From an educational perspective, the aim of the placement was not to produce experts in the treatment of alcoholism, clearly an impossible task in the allotted time, but rather to enable the students to recognise and deal appropriately with alcohol related problems which they would inevitably meet in their psychiatric and general nursing careers, and to attempt to promote positive attitudes towards alcoholism and alcoholics.

The treatment programme was very structured, consisting of formal group therapy 7 days per week over a 6-week period, and was the same for all patients. It was partly educational, partly skills based (for example, teaching assertiveness skills), and partly aimed at attitude change. In the experimental training programme, the first 6 weeks of the students' 12-week placement involved undergoing the same course of treatment as the patients, the main difference being that, for obvious reasons, the students spent only 8 hours per day on the unit instead of 24. Other than that, the experience was designed to be as close to that of the patients as possible. The students thus not only took part in group therapy, but also spent their spare time with the patients, ate with them, watched TV with them, and even spent several nights on the unit. They were immersed in the patient culture and thus, in a sense, became patients.

The students' experience might seem on first sight to be similar to that gained in a therapeutic community. However, the main difference between the situation in Ward X and that in a therapeutic community is that in the former, the staff–patient roles were well defined, whereas in the latter they blur and to some extent overlap. Furthermore, although therapeutic communities are in themselves learning situations, the students obtain their formal teaching from staff in all-staff settings, whereas in Ward X the students learnt mainly from patients in patient–staff or all-patient settings. Because the roles are so blurred in therapeutic communities, students can still identify with the staff, whereas on Ward X the students were pushed very much into the patient role, thus enabling empathy with patients to be quickly built up.

The experience was therefore more like an extended role-play exercise, or rather a series of 8-hour role-plays, since debriefing through reflective interviews took place at the end of each session. Coupled with the role-play was the opportunity to take part in group therapy as a patient rather than as a thera-pist, and the combination of the two was thought to offer not only an invaluable insight into the psychology of the alcoholic, but also a great deal of practical and theoretical knowledge about alcohol and alcoholism. It could be argued that, as the students were not themselves alcoholics, they would not benefit from the treatment programme. However, it has already been noted that T-groups are an established educational method, and research has shown that participation in group work can bring about changes in attitudes, values and self-image (Campbell and Dunnette, 1968) with an orientation towards growth and change (Lieberman *et al.*, 1973). Furthermore, these changes last a year or more before starting to fade (Mangham and Cooper, 1969).

Although the prospect of change can be exciting, and the changes themselves are clearly educationally valuable, participation in a therapeutic group is usually also threatening, not least because it highlights any shortcomings in the student. Thus:

> one major consequence... is that learners often come alive to how much they commonly miss or neglect in interpersonal and intergroup relation-ships. This realisation can be threatening for some, even intimidating. And for (apparently few) others, this realisation of how much they miss or neglect can sometimes be incapacitating. (Blumberg and Golembiewski, 1976)

For nurses who are accustomed to erecting firm barriers between themselves and their patients, there is another threat, identified by Yalom (1970):

> All accoutrements which in the outside world symbolise success and normality are deposited at the door of the T-group. Individuals are no longer rewarded for their material success, for their hierarchical position, for their unruffled aplomb, for their efficiency, or for their expertise in their area of specialisation; instead they are exposed to the totally different values of the T-group, in which they are rewarded for interpersonal honesty and for the disclosure of self-doubts and weaknesses.

Nevertheless, the anxiety produced as a result of group experiences is, according to House (1967), not only inevitable but also desirable, and change cannot occur without it. Thus, while it is important to be aware of signs of stress in students undergoing an experience of this kind, Gibb (1970) found the number of people suffering adverse effects from group experience to be only a fraction of 1 percent of the participants.

Evaluating the experience

Two third-year students took part in the experiment together, and it formed the first 6 weeks of their 12-week placement on Ward X. Immediately following their experience, an evaluation was conducted. This evaluation, which was of the experiment rather than of the students, was carried out by interview, the aim being to ascertain any change in attitudes, feelings and values, as well as to discover ways in which the experience could be improved.

One result which took everyone by surprise was the intensity of emotions experienced by the students. In particular, they reported feeling a great deal of anger, mostly directed towards the staff. However, this anger was dealt with in a positive way and accounted for much of the insight and self-awareness gained from the course:

> I've never experienced so much anger before, I really haven't, and to actually work through that, and to get over it, and to find ways of getting rid of it, is positive. I was in such an angry state that I had to be honest

for once. I must admit, I'm not a very honest person with feelings, and I was this time.

The students also gained valuable experience of group dynamics, particularly of the way in which group participation encourages self-disclosure:

> Just being part of the group, feeling part of the group, is a positive experience. A learning one as well. Now I would feel a lot more confident about running a group, and feel very sensitive to people's needs after being part of a group, 'cos you actually know what it feels like.

Empathy towards patients was expressed, and not being alcoholic was not seen as a barrier to understanding how they were feeling. Attitudes towards alcoholism and alcoholics changed considerably, and cognitive understanding increased:

> Before I came, I used to think that alcoholism was a weak minded, self inflicted illness. I don't see it as being that any more. Before I came I thought that people drank because of problems. I realise that's not true. I realise that perhaps their drinking increases due to problems for the pure fact that they cannot actually cope at that time, but I see them as just people who've been caught up in this slow, insidious process of drinking.

Weaknesses in the experiment were also identified. In particular, the students found difficulties in deroling at the end of the shift, and identified the need for a neutral person, that is someone not connected with the unit, to help with the problem. Also, although the students were told they could abandon the project at any time, they did not see the offer as being genuine, and did not want to be seen, or to see themselves, as failing:

> I don't think I had a choice, no, and that was partly coming from me, saying 'carry on'. It didn't appear genuine to me, and plus I wanted to prove to them: 'No, I'm not gonna back out, I'm gonna do it'.

As yet, the experiment has not been repeated, although there is scope for similar projects to be set up in a variety of clinical environments. Clearly, there are dangers involved, and particular care must be taken to properly debrief the students at the end of each shift. However, I believe the benefits outweigh the risks, and that a truly patient-centred placement of this kind can provide a rich and unforgettable experience which has immense value in helping students to empathise and build relationships with patients.

The first day as a patient, I thought the whole experience was going to be pretty amusing. It seemed quite fun at the time to be treated as a patient. As far as I'm concerned, I'm not ashamed of any of the feelings I've had, I'm not embarrassed by anything. I've come through six weeks and I feel great about it.

References

Blumberg, A. and Golembiewski, R.T. (1976) *Learning and Change in Groups*. Harmondsworth: Penguin.

Campbell, J.P. and Dunnette, M.D. (1968) Effectiveness of T-group experiences in managerial training and development. *Psychol. Bull.*, **70**, 73-104.

Davies, I.K. (1971) *The Management of Learning*. New York: McGraw-Hill.

Fromm, E. (1973) *The Anatomy of Human Destructiveness*. London: Cape.

Gibb, J.R. (1970) The effects of human relations in training. In: *Handbook of Psychotherapy and Behaviour Change* (A.E. Bergin and S.L. Garfield (eds). New York: John Wiley.

House, R.J. (1967) T-group education and leadership effectiveness: a review of the literature and a critical evaluation. *Person. Psychol.*, **20**, 1-32.

Lieberman, M.A., Yalom, I.D. and Miles, M.B. (1973) *Encounter Groups: First Facts*. New York: Basic Books.

Mangham, I. and Cooper, C.L. (1969) The impact of T-groups on managerial behaviour. *J. Management Studies*, **6**, 53-72.

Milgram, S. (1963) Behavioural study of obedience. *J. Abnorm. Soc. Psychol.*, **67**, 371-378.

Rogers, C.R. (1957) The necessary and sufficient conditions of therapeutic personality change. *J. Consult. Psychol.*, **21**, 95-103.

Yalom, I.D. (1970) *The Theory and Practice of Group Psychotherapy*. New York: Basic Books.

Zimbardo, P. (1972) Pathology of Imprisonment. *Trans-Action*, **9**, 4-8.

Epilogue

Progress is marked less by a perfection of consensus than by a refinement of debate. What gets better is the precision with which we vex each other

Clifford Geertz

Imagination is more important than knowledge

Albert Einstein

Nursing is now firmly embedded in a business culture, the business of healthcare. It is being seen increasingly as a commodity to be purchased, and must therefore prove its worth in terms of value for money against a variety of other forms of treatment and therapy. It is the health commissions and, indirectly, the trusts and hospitals who now hold the purse strings, and it can no longer be taken for granted that nurses are an essential part of their long-term plans for healthcare provision.

So what do the purchasers of healthcare want from nurses? On the one hand, there are suggestions of an integration of roles and a move towards a generic healthcare worker who will complement or support the role of the doctor, while on the other hand there is pressure on many nurses to take on part of the doctor's role, particularly in the light of the current crisis over junior doctors' hours. Therefore, if nursing is to survive as a viable and autonomous profession, it has to put its cards on the table. We need to say what it is that makes nursing special, what, if anything, nurses can contribute to healthcare provision that other professional groups cannot.

I have attempted to argue in this book that nursing is different and separate from medicine, that it is concerned with holistic care, with healing rather than with curing. The problem is, of course, that in a market-driven healthcare system, these aims and outcomes are not often seen as important, and arguably the main reason for this is not because they are not valid or useful outcomes, but because they are difficult to measure.

And of course the reason why measurement is so important is not a concern with quality of care, but with having a point of comparison in what is rapidly becoming an extremely competitive market. Customers, whether they are fundholding GP practices or individual patients, are being encouraged to make purchasing choices, and it is therefore necessary that they have some kind of criteria on which to base their decisions.

I am reluctant, however, to jump onto the user-movement, customer-is-always-right bandwagon, because the customer is only always right when all we are concerned with is taking his money. Of course it is important to listen to what the customer (although for reasons given in the Preface, I prefer the term patient) is saying and to involve him in decision making, but my belief is that we should be listening to our own patients (and for those of us in education, to our own students) as individuals rather than relying on large-scale, macro surveys to inform us of what our patients and students *en masse* want from us.

There are two reasons why that approach is flawed. The first has been the subject of a large part of this book, and concerns the inability of macro social research to tell us anything about specific individuals. At best, such an approach can only result in a crude utilitarianism based on the greatest good for the greatest number, in which minority views are swallowed up in the process of statistical analysis.

But a second and more compelling reason is that a macro approach to customer satisfaction inevitably leads to measuring not what is important but what is measurable. We are therefore witnessing a growing reductionist trend towards defining quality as what can be determined by crude, quantitative indicators such as bed occupancy, patient throughput and out-patient waiting times, and the danger, which is fast becoming a reality, is that nursing effectiveness will be assessed in these terms.

However, I believe that asking whether nursing can have an impact on these variables is to ask the wrong question, and I maintain that we should be saying so as a profession, and saying so loudly. Of course waiting time is an important factor, but it is not the most important factor, and it should not be the concern of nurses. The health service employs large numbers of accountants and computer programmers, but nobody judges them on whether they reduce bed occupancy or whether they increase the flow of patients through the system, and the same should be true of nurses. Furthermore, I suspect that the Government's focus on such irrelevances as the Patients' Charter and the Health of the Nation targets is a smokescreen to distract us from the real issues such as the failure of the care in the community initiative, the growing disillusionment of many healthcare workers, and the ongoing programme of hospital closures due to lack of cash.

Nursing interventions are concerned with quality of care, not quantity, and I do not believe that we should be drawn into justifying nursing care in terms of quantitative measures. Indeed, I see the task of the nursing profession not as attempting to provide what the purchasers are requesting, but rather as attempting to persuade the purchasers to request what nurses are, or should be, providing. The customer is not always right. In fact he is frequently wrong, no matter how many millions of pounds he holds in his budget. As Bob Dylan put it, money doesn't speak, it swears.

The problem, of course, is that real quality of care, and indeed quality of life, is an extremely elusive concept, but we must not be seduced into thinking that because something is unmeasurable that it is therefore unimportant. In fact, the opposite is probably true; the more important and relevant a concept, the more difficult it is to pin it down and measure it.

So, if what nurses do is not only unmeasurable, but also undefinable, how can they market it? In order to answer that question, we must return to a concept that has been one of the foundation stones of this book, and that is the notion of process as opposed to content or outcome. If nursing is to sell itself on the strength of what it produces, then not only does it run up against the problem of not having a readily identifiable product, but also it might well find itself squeezed out of the market by the technical skills and knowledge of the medical profession on one side, and the low cost of healthcare support workers on the other. And to attempt to compete with either, by becoming more medically and technically oriented or by selling itself more cheaply, is, I maintain, professional suicide.

No, what is unique about nursing, particularly patient-centred, primary nursing, is the process rather than the outcome. In the words of the song, it's not what you do, it's the way that you do it, and nursing's way is through the therapeutic relationship. And the therapeutic relationship, as I hope this book has demonstrated, is not simply a process of befriending or being with a patient, but a highly skilled and specialised activity which unites practice, research and education in the indivisible whole of nursing praxis.

Praxis therefore complements rather than challenges the medical profession. Whereas the macro approach of medicine paints in broad brush strokes and primary colours, the micro, patient-centred approach of praxis fills in the details and expands the range of hues. Medical and social research tells us how to treat and care for people in general, the greatest good for the greatest number; praxis tells us how to treat and care for each unique individual. Thus, in many cases, praxis is more concerned with when not to treat than it is with when to treat. The doctor might prescribe the new wonder drug which has been found in clinical trials to be effective in 99 per cent of all cases, but the nurse–practitioner will know the one case in a hundred when it should not be given, simply because she knows her patients intimately as people rather than as statistics. And as I have pointed out, this knowing goes far beyond the social. It is founded on a deep therapeutic relationship and a scientific process of coming to understand patients as dynamic, biopsychosocial systems on the one hand, and as unique individual persons on the other.

The foundations of nursing praxis have already been laid, and date back at least to the work of Hildegard Peplau in the 1950s, and possibly right back to Nightingale herself. The challenge for those of us in education and research, those of us who define and maintain the dominant nursing paradigm, is therefore to listen to what our practice colleagues are telling us, and to work together to promote and consolidate a new paradigm for nursing which will carry us into the twenty-first century.

Glossary

If I don't know I don't know, I think I know
If I don't know I know, I think I don't know

R.D. Laing

Disputation is a proof of not seeing clearly

Chuang Tzu

Abduction/abductive reasoning   A form of logical reasoning usually associated with American philosopher Charles Pierce, which attempts to explain single events from a combination of personal knowledge and generalisable theory.

Action research   An approach to doing research which aims to bring about change in the situation being investigated as a direct result of carrying out the research.

Aesthetic knowledge   A term coined by Carper to describe knowledge which is individual, particular and unique, and which enables us to go beyond what can be explained by empirical scientific knowledge.

Anti-positivist   See *Interpretive.*

Co-operative inquiry   An approach to doing research which breaks down the barriers between researcher and subject, and which sees research as being carried out with or for people rather than on them.

Critical incident analysis   A form of *reflective practice* in which a practitioner explores specific incidents of particular importance or significance.

Deduction/deductive reasoning   A form of logical reasoning in which information about particular cases is deduced from general statements of fact.

Empirical knowledge   Objective, publicly verifiable knowledge derived through the senses.

Epistemology   A branch of philosophy concerned with the nature of knowledge and claims about knowledge.

Erklären   A German word meaning 'explanation' which was adopted by Weber as characterising the aim of the natural sciences in contrast to *Verstehen*.

Formal theory   A term employed by Usher and Bryant to describe generalisable scientific theory, in contrast to *informal theory*.

Free group discussion   An educational technique described by Abercrombie in which students discuss pre-examined material in small groups.

Hypothesising   Part of the process of *reflexive practice* in which hypotheses about individual patients are formulated and tested out in clinical situations.

Hypothetico-abductivism   An alternative to the scientific methods of *inductivism* and *hypothetico-deductivism* for generating knowledge and informing practice in individual nurse–patient situations.

Hypothetico-deductivism   A scientific method proposed by Popper as an alternative to *inductivism*, in which scientists attempt to disprove fully formed generalisable hypotheses.

Induction/inductive reasoning   A form of logical reasoning in which a number of individual cases are employed in order to induce a generalisable statement of fact.

Inductivism   A scientific method based on *inductive reasoning* in which a finite number of individual observations are generalised into a global theory.

Informal model   A term employed in this book to describe a framework or process for constructing *informal theory.*

Informal theory   Personal theory about unique and specific situations which is not generalisable beyond those situations, in contrast to *formal theory* which is public and generalisable.

Interpretive   Subjective, mainly qualitative school of social research in contrast to the *positivist* school.

Knowing how   Practical, experiential knowledge which is unique to individual practitioners, in contrast to *knowing that*.

Knowing that   Theoretical, publicly obtainable textbook knowledge, in contrast to *knowing how*.

Level 1 research   A term used in this book to describe research which is concerned with generating usually quantitative data for others to interpret.

Level 2 research   Research whose aim is to analyse and interpret data for others to apply to practical situations.

Level 3 research   Research which is concerned with the generation of *personal knowledge* and *informal, micro theory*, usually through the process of *reflection-on-action*.

Level 4 research   Research whose aim is to bring about change in practice as part of doing the research, and in which the change *reflexively* modifies the research process.

Macro theory/understanding   Theory based on the statistical behaviour of large numbers, in contrast to *micro theory*.

Methodological pluralism   An eclectic and pragmatic approach to research common in nursing, which employs a variety of qualitative and quantitative methods.

Micro theory/understanding   Theory based on an understanding of individual cases, in contrast to *macro theory*.

Normal science   A term used by Kuhn to denote a period of stability and consolidation in a discipline, in contrast to scientific revolution.

Nurse-practitioner   A term employed in this book to describe a nurse who generates her own *informal theory* out of practice through *reflection-in-action*, in contrast to the *nurse-technician*.

Nurse–technician　A term employed in this book to describe a nurse who applies knowledge and theories generated by researchers and academics, in contrast to the *nurse–practitioner*.

Nursing models　A term used to describe a conceptual representation of a nursing theory, or sometimes as an alternative term for the theory itself.

Nursing praxis　A term employed in this book to describe a model which integrates *reflection-on-action, reflection-in-action, formal theory* and *informal theory* through the process of *hypothetico-abductivism*.

On-the-spot experimenting　Another name for *reflection-in-action*.

Paradigm　A shared set of rules and beliefs about how a discipline functions, including what counts as knowledge, how it can be generated, and how and by whom it can be disseminated.

Paradigm case　A term used by Benner to denote a powerful and memorable experience which can be employed to inform future practice.

Personal knowledge　A body of knowledge relating to individual cases from practice which is unique to its holder and can often not be put into words.

Positivist　Objective, mainly quantitative school of research which generates empirical knowledge through the application of formal scientific method.

Post-technocratic education　A term used by Bines to refer to a model of education which recognises *personal knowledge* and *informal theory* as valid forms of knowing.

Practicum　A practice setting which simulates the real world, but is relatively free of its pressures, distractions, and risks.

Practitioner-based inquiry/research　A form of research in which practitioners explore their own practice using *reflective* and *reflexive* techniques.

Praxis　A Greek term to denote the coming together of theory and practice as a single and indivisible whole. See also *Nursing praxis*.

Pre-technocratic education An apprenticeship model of education in which instruction takes place mainly on the job, but which might also include block or day release in a classroom setting.

Problem of deduction A term used in this book for the problem in nursing of attempting to apply generalisable *macro theories* based on statistical data to individual cases.

Problem of induction A problem of the scientific method of *inductivism* that no amount of observations of individual cases can ever prove a global, generalisable *macro theory*.

Problem of verification A term used in this book for a problem of the scientific method of *hypothetico-deductivism* that no amount of testing ever verifies a *macro theory*.

Reflection-in-action A term used by Schön for reflection in the practice setting whilst still engaged in practice, with the aim that the reflection will be immediately employed to reflexively shape and modify that practice. See also *On-the-spot experimenting*.

Reflection-on-action A term employed by Schön for the retrospective contemplation of practice, usually away from the setting in which the practice took place.

Reflective education An educational process which encourages and facilitates *reflection-on-action* as a means of generating knowledge and theory out of practice.

Reflective practice The process of reflecting on or in practice.

Reflective practicum A clinical setting in which students are facilitated to generate new, *personal knowledge* and test out informal theory.

Reflective research See *Level 3 research*.

Reflective spiral curriculum A curriculum model based on Kolb's reflective learning cycle, in which students are facilitated to generate *personal knowledge* and *informal theory* at ever deeper and more personal levels.

Reflexive education An educational process which aims to develop *nursing praxis* by facilitating the student to build and modify theory and practice during the therapeutic encounter through *reflection-in-action*.

Reflexive practice   See *Nursing praxis.*

Reflexive research   See *Level 4 research.*

Situational repertoire   A personal store of *paradigm cases* employed in *reflective practice.*

Student-centred learning   A term used by Carl Rogers to describe a philosophy of education in which the students exert some control over the content and process of the learning experience.

Tacit knowledge   A term employed by Polanyi for personal, practical knowledge that cannot easily be put into words or described to others.

Technical rationality   A term used by Schön to describe the hierarchical relationship between traditional science and its practical application.

Technocratic education   A model of education based on *technical rationality* in which pure science is taught first, and is then applied to practical situations.

Theory-practice gap   The gap, particularly noticeable in nursing, between what theory and research says ought to happen in practice, and what actually does happen.

Verstehen   A German word meaning 'understanding' which was adopted by Weber as characterising the aim and methods of the social sciences in contrast to *Erklären.*

World 2 knowledge   A term used by Popper to describe the body of personal knowledge that each of us carries around in our head.

World 3 knowledge   A term used by Popper to describe objective, public knowledge to be found in books, journals and other media.

Short reading list

We feel that even when all possible scientific questions have been answered, the problems of life remain completely untouched

Ludwig Wittgenstein

The philosophers have only interpreted the world, in various ways; the point, however, is to change it.

Karl Marx

Introduction

This list is for readers who would like to follow up some of the ideas presented in the book. Some aspects of the new paradigm are based on nursing theory and practice, but much of it is drawn from writers in other fields: from psychologists, from educationalists and from philosophers, and the reading list reflects this mix. However, when books from other disciplines have been cited, often all the reader needs to do is to substitute the word 'nursing' for 'education', 'psychology' or whatever throughout, and the book will make perfect sense (for example, Altrichter *et al*.). Additionally, some of the books on the list are primary sources (for example, Schön) and some are summaries or reviews of the literature (for example, Hart and Bond).

For convenience, the reading has been divided into four sections of theory, practice, research and education, which reflects the structure of this book. However, this is to some extent an artificial distinction, and some of the books attempt an integration of the four sections (for example, Usher and Bryant, which although written for teachers, is easily transferable to nursing). Also, by restricting myself to five books from each section, what emerges is a somewhat arbitrary 'top twenty' from which some very useful books were, out of necessity, omitted.

None of these books, however, will make you a better practitioner (including the one you are now reading), and words are no substitute for action. As this book has tried to argue, the most important theory for nurse–practitioners is the theory that they generate for themselves from their own practice, and so ultimately, if this book has a message, it is that the only book that will really influence your practice is the one you write yourself.

Theory

Capra, F. (1982) *The Turning Point*. New York: Simon and Schuster.
Garnham, A. and Oakhill, J. (1994) *Thinking and Reasoning*. Oxford: Blackwell.
Hollis, M. (1994) *The Philosophy of Social Science*. Cambridge: Cambridge University Press.
Usher, R. and Bryant, I. (1989) *Adult Education as Theory, Practice and Research*. London: Routledge.
Ziman, J. (1978) *Reliable Knowledge*. Cambridge: Cambridge University Press.

Practice

Benner, P. (1984) *From Novice to Expert*. California: Addison-Wesley.
Palmer, A., Burns, S. and Bulman, C. (1994) *Reflective Practice in Nursing*. Oxford: Blackwell Scientific.
Pearson, A. (1988) *Primary Nursing*. London: Croom Helm.
Peplau, H.E. (1952) *Interpersonal Relationships in Nursing*. Basingstoke: Macmillan.
Schön, D.A. (1983) *The Reflective Practitioner*. London: Temple Smith.

Research

Altrichter, H., Posch, P. and Somekh, B. (1993) *Teachers Investigate their Work*. London: Routledge.

Cassell, C. and Symon, G. (1994) *Qualitative Methods in Organizational Research*. London: Sage.

Hart, E. and Bond, M. (1995) *Action Research for Health and Social Care*. Buckingham: Open University Press.

McNiff, J. (1993) *Teaching as Learning*. London: Routledge.

Reason, P. (1988) *Human Inquiry in Action*. London: Sage.

Education

Bines, H. and Watson, D. (eds) (1992) *Developing Professional Education*. Buckingham: Open University Press.

Carr, W. and Kemmis, S. (1986) *Becoming Critical*. London: Falmer Press.

Gibbs, G. (1992) *Improving the Quality of Student Learning*. Bristol: Technical and Educational Services.

Rogers, C. (1983) *Freedom to Learn for the 80s*. Ohio: Merrill.

Stenhouse, L. (1975) *An Introduction to Curriculum Research and Development*. Oxford: Heinemann.

Index